AROMATHERAPY
for the SOUL

Also by
Valerie Ann Worwood

AROMATHERAPY FOR THE HEALTHY CHILD

THE COMPLETE BOOK OF
ESSENTIAL OILS & AROMATHERAPY

ESSENTIAL AROMATHERAPY
(WITH SUSAN WORWOOD)

THE FRAGRANT MIND

SCENTS & SCENTUALITY

AROMATHERAPY
for the SOUL

Healing the Spirit with Fragrance and Essential Oils

VALERIE ANN WORWOOD

NEW WORLD LIBRARY
NOVATO, CALIFORNIA

New World Library
14 Pamaron Way
Novato, California 94949

© 1999 Valerie Ann Worwood

Published in 1999 by New World Library as *The Fragrant Heavens*

The material in this book is not meant to take the place of professional spiritual
guidance or medical diagnosis and treatment by a qualified medical practitioner. All
recommendations herein contained are believed to be effective, but since actual use of
essential oils by others is beyond the author's and publisher's control, no expressed or
implied guarantee as to the effects of their use can be given nor liability taken.

Text layout and design by Margaret Copeland, Terragraphics
Illustrations on page 300 by Edwina Hammin

Library of Congress Cataloging-in-Publication Data
Worwood, Valerie Ann
Aromatherapy for the soul : healing the spirit with fragrance and essential oils / by
Valerie Ann Worwood.
    p.   cm.
Includes bibliographical references and index.
1. Aromatherapy. 2. Spiritualism. I. Title.
RM666.A68W677   1998   98-22936
615'.321—dc21

First printing of *Aromatherapy for the Soul*, September 2006
Printed in Canada on acid-free, partially recycled paper
ISBN-10: 1-57731-562-6
ISBN-13: 978-1-57731-562-9
Distributed by Publishers Group West

10 9 8 7 6

For Nan and Pop, who reminded me that "there are more things between heaven and earth than we will ever know about," and Uncle Will, who understood the spiritual importance of fragrant plants.

There are eighty myriads of trees in every corner of Paradise, the meanest among them choicer than all the spice trees. In every corner there are sixty myriads of angels singing with sweet voices, and the tree of life stands in the middle and shades the whole of Paradise. It has fifteen thousand tastes, each different from the other, and the perfumes thereof vary likewise. Over it hang seven clouds of glory, and winds blow upon it from all sides, so that its odor is wafted from one end of the world to the other.

— Louis Ginzberg, *Legends of the Bible*

Contents

PART TWO: AROMATHERAPY AND
THE SPIRITUAL CONNECTION

Charts and Illustrations

Chapter 8: Multidimensional Bodies

Chapter 9: Vibrational Aromatherapy

Chapter 10: Energetic Aromatherapy

Chapter 12: The Aromatic Traditions

Introduction

To see a World in a Grain of Sand
And a Heaven in a Wild Flower,
Hold Infinity in the palm of your hand
And Eternity in an hour.
        — William Blake,
        Auguries of Innocence

THE OMNIPRESENT DIVINE has been put through the prism of human experience, and is expressed in many different ways. Some people focus their ideas of the Divine on an original creator, God, and venerate prophets of that God. Some spiritual traditions pay reverence to the whole living environment, paying respect to the vast landscape and all that lives and grows on it. Others turn more inward and use specific mental exercises to connect with the oneness of the universe. Whether we pray to God, whether we pay homage to Mother Earth, Father Sky, or the spirit of the sage, whether we look to the stars, or seek the stars within, spirituality is about making connections. We may take different routes, but the destination is the same.

Although spiritual practices differ greatly, it's no coincidence that so many use fragrance. Every evening in India, the air is rich with the aroma of incense burning at home shrines. Smoke fragrant with the aroma of the smoldering resins, frankincense and myrrh, fills the air in Ethiopian Coptic and Orthodox Christian churches. Muslims use lavish quantities of sweet-smelling rose water to impart fragrance to mosques and other holy places. In Native American sweat lodges, for ritual purification and spiritual connection, the fragrant herbs of sage, cedar, and sweetgrass are put on the hot rocks to release their aroma molecules into the humid atmosphere. Clouds of fragrant smoke rise from handfuls of incense sticks, placed at Chinese Buddhist shrines. In the habdalah ceremony in Jewish homes at the close of the Sabbath every Saturday night, blessings for light and fragrance are recited over the candle and spice box. Each dawn, Tibetans go up on the roofs of their houses and light stoves in which they burn bundles of juniper — to force the sky door open. As plumes of smoke rise from the houses and fragrance fills the air, prayers can be heard.

It's the essential oils in fragrant plant materials, the aroma molecules, that are released by these various practices — they are what gives incense its aroma, just as it's the essential oil in pine needles that gives a pine forest its uplifting quality. Essential oils exude from plants into their "headspace," where we smell them when walking among nature, and humans have devised many methods to capture this essence of the plant, the molecules so many people have chosen to help them connect with and feel the Divine.

Fragrance has been said to alert the gods to our presence, and act as a sign that the human mind is focused and receptive to spiritual guidance. In many cultures sweet-smelling aromas were and still are associated with divinity — with gods, heavens, angels, and saints all being attributed with having a delightful fragrance. By oneself being fragrant or burning fragrant material, a link or bridge could be formed to the Divine. In *Legends of the Bible*, Louis Ginzberg tells us that the Tabernacle had two altars: one brass, and used for food offerings, corresponding to the body; and one of gold, used for offering spices and sweet incense — "for the soul takes delight in perfumes only."

Many reasons have been given for the use of fragrance for spiritual assistance, but what's equally interesting is the sheer endurance of the practice. It's not an old habit that's dying out. On the contrary, as well as continuing in the older spiritual traditions, fragrance is being used also by the new. As I travel and visit places and people, I can see fragrant oils being used in all kinds of contexts, including different forms of healing, counseling, prayer, and meditation.

Fragrance and spirituality mingle as one in the spiritual traditions of the world. The heavens are redolent with exquisite aromas, the gods are sweetly fragrant, as are angels, saints, and those touched by the Divine. The odor of sanctity has impressed many nations, and the people, in turn, make offerings of sweet-smelling fragrant aroma to the deity.

The Polynesian god Urutaete carried souls of the dead to Rohutu noanoa, a garden paradise perfumed with exquisite odors, known as "Fragrant Rohutu" or "Perfumed Rohutu." Buddhists will pass to the fragrant mountain known as "gandhamadana." The gods of the ancient Greeks lived on the fragranced Mount Olympus, while Elysium, the pre-Hellenic paradise, was reserved for human heroes and heroines. They passed there without dying, and found the Elysian fields suffused with delicious aroma. According to Homer, those favored by the gods had their body and soul made immortal in this land of perfect happiness. Lucian spoke of the "scented Isles of the Blessed," and a golden city beside a river of myrrh; while Plutarch wrote about the intoxicating fragrance rising from the River Lethe where "souls were imbibing these delicious scents aglow with pleasure and engaging in concourse with the other."

The exhalations of the Muslim Paradise have been described as of "musk, ginger, amber, and from the very ground of Eden. The French Christian saint Gregor, around 580 CE, apparently after a brief sojourn there, said paradise was a "prairie from which rises at all times an extraordinary perfume."

In the last book of the New Testament, Revelation 5:8, we hear of the twenty-four elders in heaven who fell down before the Lamb "having every one of them harps, and golden vials full of odors, which are the prayers of saints." Heaven is fragrant indeed. In Revelation 8:3, an angel came to the altar, holding a golden censer and was given much incense "that he should offer it with the prayers of all saints upon the golden altar which was before the throne. And the smoke of the incense . . . ascended up before God."

The presence of the Holy Spirit is often said to be made known by a mystical fragrance, while so many Christian saints were said to be sweet smelling or to produce fragrant relics that the idea of an "odor of sanctity" has likewise continued through the aeons of time. Homer described the Greek god Zeus as "wreathed in a fragrant cloud," and the ancient Greeks and Romans recognized they were in the presence of a deity when they smelled a specially powerful fragrant odor. Artemis appeared in this way, as did Bacchus — who smelled of saffron and myrrh. The garments of Demeter were said to be fragrant, while Aphrodite/Venus had fragrant robes and hair, and a fragrant temple. Plato wrote of Eros, "Love will not settle on body or soul or aught else that is flowerless or whose flower has faded away."

Gods were often said to have been born from various scented parts of plants — the resin that exuded from a cut in a tree, the fragrant bark that was so often used for making incense, or a flower that was, or still is, used for making perfume. The ancient Egyptian god Amon Ra emerged from a lotus, as did the Indian god Brahma, while Adonis was born from a myrrh tree. The Egyptians called the incense resin that exuded from certain trees, "the tears" or "sweat" of the gods.

Egyptian hieroglyphics tell the story of the holy conception of Queen Hatshepsut. Her mother, Queen Ahmose, was awakened from her sleep in her beautiful palace by the majestic aroma of the god Amon. "All his odors were from Punt," the inscription says, which is perhaps why his daughter, Hatshepsut, felt driven to organize a trade delegation to the land of Punt (probably present-day Somalia) with orders to bring back an incense tree, which she had planted in the garden in front of her palace.

Shamans across the world today, as ever, use fragrance to invite the ancestral, animal, or nature spirits into this world, and sometimes spirits are recognized as being present by their fragrance alone. So it is with the Chewong of the Malay Peninsula, who have a group of female spirits they call the "leaf people" — they are recognized by non-shamans as being present in the meeting house only by their fragrance. Nearby, the Batek Negrito say their spirits live in a land that is perpetually fragrant with the aroma of fruit blossoms, and that they love incense and the scent of flowers, while the Warao of Venezuela believe that fragrance originated in the refreshing land of the God of Life.

Places of worship were often fragrant because of the building material used. The temple of Solomon where Jesus taught in Jerusalem was made with the magnificent, fragrant cedars that once covered Lebanon. Indian sandalwood temples are called *gandhakuti*, meaning "houses of fragrance," and at the Spiritual Grove Temple in Hangzhou, China, an aromatic effigy of Buddha stands fifty feet tall and emits the aroma of its seventy-four blocks of camphor wood.

When the Dalai Lama was a young boy, Tibetans still walked, and prostrated themselves on the earth, along the circuitous processional route to the monastery at Lhasa, past endless fires of burning juniper. Today, sadly as refugees in Ladakh, Kashmir, the Drokpa Tibetans in particular burn huge amounts of juniper in offering to the minor deities and gods of place — a tradition that predates Buddhism and denotes purification, atonement, and hope for rebirth.

The long aromatic tradition is often hidden in symbols, the origins of which we have long since ceased to question. The word *rosary*, for example, stems from the fact that early Christian priests wore garlands of roses around their necks on feast days. The first rosaries were made from 165 rosebuds or rolled-up rose petals, sometimes held in place with lampblack. And the famous Jewish candlestick with seven arms, the menorah, the emblem of Israel for over three thousand years, is a material replica of the fragrant healing plants of the *Salvia* species that not long ago covered Mount Moriah in Jerusalem.

At Jesus' birth, the kings brought gifts of gold, frankincense, and myrrh — gold, perhaps, to help financially, frankincense and myrrh as incense material and medicine. Two days before the Crucifixion, Mary Magdalen took "a pound of ointment of spikenard, very costly, and anointed the feet of Jesus, and wiped his feet with her hair, and the house was filled with the odor of the ointment" (John 12:3–7). Spikenard is related to the valerian plant; its aroma is earthy yet sweet, and its effect is sedative. Jesus was going to need it, and when Judas Iscariot complained at the waste of such a quantity of precious oil, saying the three hundred pence it cost could be given to the poor, Jesus said, "Let her alone: against the day of my burying hath she kept this" (John 12:7).

The word *messiah* means "the anointed one." Kings had from very early times been anointed as a sign of their kingship, and Jesus was a king in the line of David. Shakespeare described the spiritual and irreversible nature of the anointing of Richard II: "Not all the water in the rough rude sea / Can wash the balm from an anointed king / The breath of worldly men cannot depose / The deputy elected of the Lord."

The ingredients of the royal anointing oil have changed little over hundreds of years. At the coronation of Queen Elizabeth II, in June 1953, it was composed of the essential oils of neroli, rose, cinnamon, and jasmine, together with benzoin, musk, civet, and ambergris, blended in sesame oil. This differs from the oil used at the coronation of Charles I in 1626, only in that sesame replaced "oil of been." Charles was anointed on the breast, between the shoulders, on both shoulders, in the angles of both arms, and on the head — seven places in all. Elizabeth was anointed on the palms, the breast, and on the head.

The coronation oil has historically been prepared by the royal physicians, in 1953 by the surgeon-apothecary, but it is applied in a spiritual context. The oils for anointing Elizabeth was consecrated — set apart as sacred to God — by the bishop of Gloucester in the chapel of St. Edward the Confessor, in Westminster Abbey, before it was laid on the altar, with the crown, ready for the ceremony. It was contained in a gold ampulla in the shape of an eagle, which was used at the coronation of Henry IV in 1399. The precious holy oil poured from the beak of the eagle into an elaborate golden spoon dating from around 1200, which, with the ampulla, is now in the crown jewels at the Tower of London. The act of anointing hallowed and dedicated Queen Elizabeth II in her office — it set the seal of God's approval.

The first English king to be anointed was Egforth of Mercia, in 785, in a ceremony derived from the Jewish tradition described in the Old Testament. The aromatic traditions go far back in time, and are continuing into the future throughout the world. Until recently we did not require an explanation as to why aroma was used in spiritual practice. Fragrance simply drifted between supplicant and deity, joining the two by the shared olfactory experience. A connection was made, and more hoped for. Today we want to know how everything works, including the spiritual use of fragrance.

Unfortunately, we have yet to figure out exactly how aroma works. We can see that two olfactory bulbs protrude from the front of the brain and have nerves extending down into the top of the nose, where they come into contact with aroma molecules. We also know that aroma is made up of molecules with particular configuration, vibration, and light-refraction qualities, and that they "lock" with receptors, sending messages to the brain. Aroma evokes memory and we can identify the part of the brain involved, but nobody has any idea how the aroma of jasmine, say, can make a picture of a garden on a warm starlit night jump into your head.

Bliss, superconsciousness, and even transcendence may prove easier to explain, as opiate and other interesting receptors are most highly concentrated in the limbic system, which is the part of the brain immediately stimulated into action by aroma molecules. Aroma molecules get as close to the brain as it is possible to get without actually *being* the brain. They stimulate the brain — that is their job — and the olfactory bulbs reach out to meet them.

Aroma evokes emotions, as well as memory, and often the two are connected. Emotions run deep, to the very core of our being. But aroma can reach them, instantaneously. Time means nothing to aroma. Although aromatic functioning is so often accidental and unconscious, within a spiritual context it is deliberate and conscious. We choose particular fragrant materials, and use them in a particular way.

The fragrance molecules, the essential oils, come from plants, to which people are inextricably linked. Plants make the air we breathe and provide the food for all living beings, on land or in water. Without them life comes to a stop. Because of them, we live, which is the humble relationship we truly have with them. We think we know about plants, and even fiddle with their genes. But the fact is, we could not *make* one plant cell from scratch. We can clone, but not create nature — because we don't know how it works. From an energetic and informational point of view, there is more to life than we know.

Essential oils contain this mystery of life; they have powerful inexplicable energies too. Standing in an ancient forest, under a thick canopy of stars, I have felt the energy of the universe. Plants are the interface between cosmic energies and the earth, upon which we depend. They capture the sun in photosynthesis; that much we know. Their aura can be caught by Kirlian photography, and even when a leaf has been cut, the otherwise invisible outline remains. What this energy is, we do not know, but we see it also emanating from humans. Here is an energy field that connects us, and the likelihood is, it is one of many.

If nature has not yet been fully explained, nor aroma, how can we hope for science to pin down spirituality? And do we even need it to? Spirituality has its own "proof" in experience. And if the scientific secret of spirituality *is* to be "discovered," it will probably be through the experience of it!

Twenty years ago in aromatherapy, there was an unwritten rule that we would not be open about the spiritual side of the essential oils we worked with. We talked about their anti-infectious qualities and their beautifying effects on the skin, or about any number of benefits to body and mind. The positive spiritual changes were recognized, but silently. It seemed far too bold to suggest the strength and confidence of nature was carried in the essential oils, or that the light and wisdom of the universe flowed through them, their fragrance like messengers from heaven, aromatic angels that come and touch us with the positivity and love of the deity.

All this is a long way from "antibacterial agents." But being able to talk about spirituality has gone hand in hand with scientific developments that have forced us to open our minds. Quantum physics and chaos theory turn everything topsy-turvy, while the insistence of physicists that the influence of an observer must be put into the experimental equation really focuses the mind. It seems the flutter of a butterfly wing on one side of the world affects events on the other side, and that what we think makes a difference to the universe. The division between body and mind has been put well and truly to rest by the latest discoveries in psychoneuroimmunoendocrinology — it appears that because there are receptors to brain chemicals throughout the whole body, mind and body are in fact one. On a molecular level, there are striking similarities between parts of humans and plants, and we can see our evolution is deeply entwined. So many connections can now be made, between people and plants, mind and body, the observer and the observed, that it is difficult to see sharp divisions. Indeed, it's now logical to state, "All is One," or agree with the inscription found on the first known picture of a distillation unit, from second-century Alexandria: "It is toward oneness that all phenomena tend."

We all have spiritual experiences; it's a question of degree. We all love, and as they say, "God is love." Love transcends time and place, so we feel that loving connection whether the loved one is with us or not. Some people hear the forest sing and are moved to their very core. Others stand in their garden in the morning and feel the unity of the universe in every shaking leaf.

Many people have had instant spiritual experiences that change their lives forever. Whatever form it takes, it is the depth and strength of the spiritual experience that carries conviction forward. More than just "tradition," spirituality puts us in touch with the cosmic network, which permeates all time and space.

From a brain biochemistry point of view, the pursuit of spirituality through aroma makes a great deal of sense, as the mechanics of smell are but one short biological step away from consciousness, including higher consciousness. Thinking of it in terms of light, essential oils *are* captured light, passed from the heavens, by plants, to us. From a vibrational, electromagnetic, and energetic point of view, essential oils *are* in harmony with life. They resonate with us, as the vibration in one violin string can cause vibration in another. We hear the message they have to bring. On a molecular level, natural plant aroma molecules touch receptors on cells with the lightest of contact, then retreat, their job of instigating a series of reactions having been done.

With an etheric quality, essential oils activate the receptors of love, compassion, and empathy. They are an informational network, carrying messages and crossing boundaries, operating on many different levels. Through them, we can contact the wisdom of nature, the power of light, the energy of the universe, and the love in our hearts.

Healing takes place on all levels — spiritual, mental, and physical, and what's so remarkable about essential oils is that they influence the whole being. Just as they are the catalyst that can make a wound heal, or a mind relax, so can they transport a soul. I know of no other substances that can do that. They are flexible, adaptable, multifaceted, deep, complex, light, subtle, etheric, and all in a positive way. If molecules could be angels, they would surely be essential oils.

The fragrant molecules that are essential oils have been the vehicles for many spiritual journeys. Weaving in and out of the body, as they weave silently through the atmosphere, ethereal but real and deep, essential oils can put us on a wavelength, a network, a web, something that connects the whole. It may be that the experience is brief, but it is never forgotten. Indeed, it is imprinted on the very soul.

Journeys often need guides, and *Aromatherapy for the Soul* is such a guide — to the spiritual aromatic adventure. I will point out landmarks, introduce aromas, and show the view. I can even take you to visit "museums of spiritual aroma" and to futuristic research labs. Beyond that, I cannot go, because spirituality is always a personal journey.

Part One

On the Celestial Wings of Fragrance

Chapter 1

Let There Be Light:
Plants and Their Spiritual Nature

As EACH DAY DAWNS, pure sunlight sparkles in dewdrops, shimmering on the grass, and on the leaves and flowers of the world. As we walk through the woods, light filters through the leaves, creating a green haven of peace. The plant world is just full of beautiful sights; there isn't a tree or flower that doesn't radiate beauty.

However, providing aesthetic pleasure is not the most important function of plants. By taking carbon dioxide and water from the air and, with light, converting it into carbohydrates, plants are the ultimate production machine, purifying the air and providing food and medicine for humans and animals, even ultimately for carnivores. Plants are both the lungs and the larder of the earth. They are the conduit between the light of the heavens and the dark of the earth, channeling energy from the sky above into the crystalline structures of Mother Earth.

Plants are magnificent. The tallest tree in Redwood National Park, California, is over 368 feet high; redwoods can live to be almost four thousand years old. The size and longevity of these masterpieces of creation are humbling, but to actually walk among the immense trees of an ancient forest is more humbling still. The smallest seed is awesome in its capacity to create another plant, perfect in every detail, including providing more seeds for future generations. Plant seeds that have been found in archaeological sites and grown, thousands of years after they were dropped there, are a testament to the monumental capacity of tiny seeds to hold life.

Most of us live in a concrete jungle, not a living, breathing one. Essential oils can restore this balance somewhat, bringing the essence of plants into our homes. To understand them fully we need to reacquaint ourselves with their heritage, their source — plants in their natural habitat.

THE SINGING FOREST

The trees are the teachers of the law.
— Brooke Medicine Eagle

In the 1950s something happened in an ancient North American forest. It was so poignant it went down in folklore, but, due to the "Chinese whispers" effect over the years, there are now two versions of the story. In one, the central character is a U.S. Forest Service employee, and in the other version he is a PhD student conducting research for his thesis on the age of trees in a bristlecone pine forest. The story goes something like this . . .

The man walked deep into the forest for many days until he found a tree he thought might be the oldest. He planned to extract a sample using a core drill so he could count its rings and date it, but the drill didn't work. For some days he tried to fix it, without success. He also had a saw. He looked at the saw and he looked at the tree. He thought about the long walk back to get another core drill and about the importance of his research. He cut down the tree and dated it. It was four thousand years old — old enough to have lived through most of known human history. When Moses was a baby, this tree was already five hundred years old.

People have different relationships with nature. Some, like the man in this story, don't treat it with the respect it deserves, making it a sacrifice to the human ego. Others claim that plants have intelligence, soul, and the capacity to communicate, and would no more cut down an ancient tree than cut down a grandmother. Attitudes differ. Some people hear the forest sing, some don't.

One hundred forty million years ago, most of the Northern Hemisphere was covered in redwood and other trees. Human beings made their appearance maybe two hundred thousand years ago and have, especially in the last two hundred years, remorselessly cut the forest down. As early as 1905, American congressman William Kent and his wife, Elizabeth, recognized the potential ecological danger, and bought 295 acres of redwood forest in California and named it Muir Woods, after the conservationist John Muir. He wrote to the Kents, "You have done me great honor, and I am proud of it." To them all, we owe thanks because today Muir Woods is one of the few remaining enclaves where you can stand among these magnificent trees without hearing the sound of a distant saw, indicating that clear-cut logging is heading your way.

It is a humbling experience to stand under ancient redwood trees. In Muir Woods, I felt like a three-year-old in the presence of very large, old, and wise men with long white beards — in awe yet certain I would be completely protected. I did not want to leave their presence. Leaning on a redwood that extended too high into the sky for me to see, I felt the energy flooding into me, a cosmic river of refreshment for the soul.

I heard the drone of a distant saw, but knew in this protected forest island it must only be someone cutting deadwood and undergrowth to clear the ground. Even so, it reminded me of other areas of the world where international logging consortiums are destroying huge areas of precious forest, and I felt the overwhelming emotions of sadness and guilt. I apologized to the trees on behalf of human beings. Strange as it may seem, the trees spoke to me, directly, without voice, from their heart to mine. They conveyed to me their resignation, deep sadness, and incomprehension as to why we should want to do such things.

Having a conversation with a tree might seem like a strange thing to do, especially when you live in a large city, a long way away from trees. But when actually out among them, it seems like the most natural thing in the world to do. I can fully understand why traditional Native Americans, when planning to cut down a tree to make a totem pole or boat, asked permission and gave thanks directly to the tree making the sacrifice.

My love of trees started when I lived in Switzerland and used to take my dog for a walk in the forest late at night. When the moon and stars illuminated our path we walked on and on, for my pleasure rather than the dog's convenience, as the silence and majesty of the forest filled me with feelings of reassurance and gratitude. It was there, high in the mountains, that I first sensed the living connection between the night sky, the trees, and the earth. Many years later, in ancient redwood and cedar forests in North America, this impression was reinforced. Standing under a thick canopy of stars illuminating the sky, I sensed that trees, particularly very tall, ancient trees, in some way act as planetary antennae. The very tops of the trees seem to attract starlight and other cosmic energies to them, "earthing" those energies as they travel down through the trunks, into the roots, and earth. I also wonder if the trees don't also transmit information back into the sky, sending vibrational energy, including human thought energy, out into the cosmos. I have no scientific proof, of course, but the thought remains: These giant trees are receivers and transmitters of energy, crucial even to cosmic balance and human spiritual growth.

Anyone who studies trees knows that there is still a great deal to learn about them, especially in terms of energy and communication. Even in terms of mechanics and chemistry, an area we think we know so much about, new discoveries are being made all the time. Scientists of the British Columbia Ministry of Forests only recently found that certain tree species can share resources using an underground network of fungal threads. Seedlings of Douglas fir, paper birch, and western red cedar were subjected to carbon dioxide containing different carbon isotopes. Two years later, 10 percent of the carbon-type fed to the birch was found in the fir. Both species share a mycorrhizal fungi that created the network of threads between them, and the carbon traveled along this complex connection. Because this same fungi does not connect with cedar, its particular experimental carbon composition was unaffected. Meanwhile, in Kenya, scientists have discovered that, as well as sucking water up from the deep earth, a "substantial" amount of water is transported downward by trees, to the dry subsurface. These are fundamental discoveries about the mechanical workings of trees, an area we thought we already understood.

In British Columbia, Canada, the drive to harvest large-dimension lumber is in full gear, as logging companies race to bring down the last remaining trees before politicians accept what environmentalists have been telling them for years, and bring the harvest to an end. Standing in these forests is scary. You can hear the drone of mechanical saws and know you're standing among doomed giants. Here are these magnificent trees, silently performing crucial ecological tasks for the whole living planet, trees that have lived through so much of human history yet are helpless to stop our saws from cutting through their bases. This helplessness, coming from such powerful, massive living things, is infinitely sad. Strangely, the trees are not angry. Perhaps they mumble to themselves, "Forgive them, for they know not what they do."

With my experience of ancient and wise trees, I was intrigued when I heard about a woman living deep in a forest in British Columbia who claims to have heard the forest sing. Where the loggers cut one-thousand-year-old trees, Gladys McIntyre earns a living planting seedling trees. In June 1990, in a part of the cedarwood forest called Howser Creek, Gladys found herself thinking about the "immense verticality" of the trees when "a profound vertical alignment took place in me in response; and suddenly I felt about twelve feet tall.

I wondered for a moment if this was soulic consciousness, then I was struck in my solar plexus by an impact of sound. It grew to an upwelling, crescendoing symphony of sound, in range and tone unlike anything I had ever heard before! Emanating from the forested hillsides across the valley, it was unquestionably a great hymn of adoration, of joy in creation and praise to the creator! Words cannot possibly express the magnitude of this joyous sound, nor my absolute awe at witnessing it."

But from being a song in praise of the Creator, the song abruptly changed from "overwhelming joy to abject sorrow." Gladys writes, "My cognitive mental faculty seemed to be translating information received by my soul from that incredible presence at worship over there." It said, "Oh noble and worthy, exploiters and conquerors, have mercy, have mercy, do not end our singing, which allows the conditions necessary to all life on the planet as you know it."

Reports as powerful as this can easily be dismissed as the workings of an overactive imagination, so I went to visit Gladys to try to get closer to the truth. I found her living with her husband, Vince, deep in the forest. They grow vegetables that are exquisitely formed, massive, with a delicious, vibrant taste. Those vegetables were like something out of a Walt Disney movie! They positively vibrated and shone in pure, verdant, colorful perfection, well loved and content. Gladys is a person clearly in touch with the laws of nature, and as sane as you or I.

I came away thinking that if the forest does communicate, Gladys is the right person to hear it. But she is not the only one. In another ancient forest, a young woman and her boyfriend went to sit on a splendid mountain ridge to admire the forest view. But instead of feeling glad to be in the splendor, the girl became overcome with the feeling of panic and fear coming from the forest. Sick with anguish, she had to return home. Days passed but the sadness wouldn't leave her. The girl felt driven to return to that part of the forest, to try to understand why she had been so affected. She was horrified and stunned to discover the whole area had been clear-cut to the ground.

Although to "civilized" people, communicating with trees may sound bizarre, it's something that's been going on a very long time. Indeed, trees have long been central to spiritual culture. In ancient Egypt, the "world tree" was associated with a "sycamore," possibly the sycamore fig that gave shade to the goddess worshippers in their groves. Kabbalah, the mystical aspect of Judaism, with its Tree of Life, has traditionally been taught to men over forty while they sat under trees. In the last book of the New Testament, Revelation 22:2, we hear that the Tree of Life is in "the midst of the street" in heaven. Buddha received enlightenment while sitting under a tree. The ancient Assyrians had many tree cults, with the Tree of Life sometimes being depicted as a cedar, fir, date, or pomegranate. The Chinese associated the Tree of Life with the peach, and in later times the cassia, while in Norse mythology it was the ash. A Polynesian legend says, "Out of this magic bread-fruit tree a great goddess was made." The sacredness of trees is universal, and this may not simply be because they routinely offer up their bounty, but because they have a spirit we can feel.

PLANTS THAT FEEL AND SPEAK

When we suddenly remember to water our plants, is it because the plants send us a message across the room, "Hey, don't forget about us!" Why shouldn't they talk to us? We talk to them. People in their high-rise apartments, or in their gardens, say to their plants, "You look lovely today," or "What's up, you're looking a bit off-color," and then fuss around them, administering love and fertilizer — organic, of course. Chatting to plants is a regular occurrence, even for royalty, and some plant aficionados play them music, taking care to choose something they like.

Edward Bach, the man who invented Bach Flower Remedies, attributed certain medicinal qualities to plants because the plants themselves told him what they were. An entire Western healing system is thus based on plant communication, and it has gone on to inspire much more plant-human exploration. Meanwhile, in many indigenous cultures, it is considered wrong to become a healer without first having dreams or visions relating to the plants used to heal. In other words, the spiritual realm is seen as the source of accurate information. Cultures that are very much in touch with the earth and all that grows on it believe totally that plants have a spirit. Obviously a plant doesn't have a voice box and mouth with which to chat, so to communicate we have to get into the common space we share, the spiritual one. If you want to know what a plant can do, go to the source and ask it. To indigenous peoples, that's the logical thing to do. There are variations on this cultural theme: some people believe the spirit of the individual plant conveys the information; some believe each species of plant has a kind of overall spirit that communicates; some believe there are a variety of nature spirits; others believe it is the voice of the Creator who speaks. These are all variations on a theme: you can speak to, or through, a plant.

The Yaqui people of northwestern Mexico have an oral tradition going back four thousand years, to 2000 BCE. Around 1500 CE, because of the oppressive actions of the Spanish conquistadors, the sacred traditions had to become secret. Seven lineages were chosen to preserve them, through sacred oral and family traditions. Through many generations the sacred way of the Yaqui was kept underground, as the bullets flew overhead. Now that we are older and wiser, hopefully, the knowledge can be revealed. Indeed, it is time for us to know it.

A man who carries this knowledge, passed to him by his father and mother, is Yaqui traditional healer Cachora Guitemea, a highly respected Native American elder. It was, then, a great privilege for me to be invited to spend a few days in the Mexican desert with Cachora to learn about sacred plant medicine. We were accompanied by both our daughters and the mutual friend who introduced us. Although Cachora is more than eighty years old and has white hair, you would never guess his age — either from his appearance or from his extraordinary energy. His face is lit up with a joy that defies time. And despite his boyish love of jokes, you never forget that you are in the presence of great wisdom and positive intent.

Cachora teaches that we must respect plants. Permission must be sought from the plant before picking it, and if the plant is required for ceremonial purposes, sacred chants and mantras are said aloud, in honor of the plant or tree. All plants have souls and spirits that guard and protect the species. It is not that every individual plant has its own, but that there is a species-spirit that has a place within plant hierarchy, depending on the sacredness of the purpose the plant is put to.

Many plants also have animal spirits attached to them, says Cachora. The connection may be derived from the fact that an animal eats from the plants and thus distributes the seeds, because the animal eats smaller animal pests upon the plants, or because the animal uses the plants as food and medicine.

Cachora is quite plain about the underlying principle of healing herbs. He says that healing takes place when a person connects into the plant spirit, becoming the plant and understanding its personality. Using spirit as the method of transference, the plant's energy or healing properties are transmitted to the person. First, the spirit of a particular species has to become known, its use and purposes memorized, its strengths and weaknesses understood. Then in times of ill health, as body, mind, and spirit are one, healing can take place by calling on the spirit and taking into one's mind the spiritual essence of the plant.

Plant life must be respected and spoken to, says Cachora, for it is part of the universe, part of ourselves, part of our heritage. I understand this to mean that everyone evolved through the plant, and through the plant cycle of crystalline life. We are all part of the same consciousness pool. Getting to know plants involves looking at them closely, communicating with them with honesty, integrity, gentleness. Human thought is the greatest obstacle to plant communication. You have to get beyond thought, into empathy and feeling through focus and concentration.

On this amazing journey, I encountered a magnificent six-foot-tall white sage bush, a grandfather of the species, having seeded many generations of plants, an elder in its own right. It was so vibrant the leaves seemed to send out showers of sparks, but I was rather taken aback when the large bush bowed its body to greet us. As there was not a hint of a breeze, I turned to my friend beside me to verify what had happened, and could tell from her wide-open eyes that she had witnessed the same action! Then the sage spoke to me, in a silent block of communication, clear and precise.

There are many indigenous peoples in the world who feel the spirit in nature, and work with it. Certain themes emerge. There is the idea that some plants should not be picked because they are too sacred, that is, too old and valuable to their "tribe." Just like us, plants need their wise elders. They say you should ask a plant if it is okay to pick it. A plant may say no or it may agree, but it is respectful to explain who the plant is for, and what is wrong with the person. The plant will then know it is not being sacrificed for no good reason. There is also the general idea that the spirit of the plant is a communal one, that it is not an individual plant that has a spirit but the species as a whole. When you communicate with a plant you communicate with its species-spirit, which at the same time can be expressed as an individual. So, when I spoke to the large sage bush I spoke to the spirit of the species, but *through* the wise old bush who, from experience, happens to hold a great deal of communal species wisdom and can express more information, more clearly.

When you think about it, this is not dissimilar to the way horticulturists and gardeners view the plants in their care. Older plants have an authority that seedlings do not. Also, each species has its own character, and individuals within the species have their particular character. We speak of animals in much the same way, saying a breed of dog might be generally "good with children," but individuals within the species might be good, or not, with children in general or with a particular child.

Many Western gardeners "tune in" to their plants in essentially the same way as do native peoples. Looking at a bed of roses, next to a bed of hollyhocks, we might perceive each species to have a different emotional tone. Each looks different, grows different, has different kinetic qualities, and different characters in much the same way people do. The more species we grow, and the longer we work with them, the more our "instinct" about plants develops (as instinct develops over time when using essential oils).

The difference between our approach and indigenous peoples' is the effort we put into learning about plants. We'll spend time reading gardening books, while they will sit with a plant for hours, days even, getting to *know* it. They'll bring it little presents, in gratitude for what it offers, in respect, and to let the plant know they *care*. They go to plants as a pupil goes to a wise person, *to learn*. Western horticulturists, on the other hand, often feel that *they* are the holders of information, and that it is their job to control the plant, which they see as their property.

We know, of course, from the concept of companion gardening that plants can influence each other in terms of preventing pests and disease. This is often accomplished through scent, as aroma molecules from one plant waft over another and exert their beneficial influence. Stephen Harrod Buhner's *Sacred Plant Medicine* provides an interesting anecdote on this subject. He was sitting with a lichen called usnea, which has powerful antibiotic qualities, when suddenly the usually subtle "feeling tone" of the usnea increased in intensity. Buhner felt his "personal boundaries" dissolving, and the plant appeared as a youngish man. The plant-man told him that usnea's primary role is to keep the earth's lung system healthy, by being an antibiotic for the trees on which it grows, adding that as a by-product of this intended role, usnea can be used to treat human lung infections. Imagine how much more we could learn about plant interaction, and how many new medicines we could discover, if more of us could hear what plants have to say.

Plants are sensitive, sentient beings. There has been a great deal of research in this area, starting in 1966 with Cleve Backster, then a New York lie-detector expert working for law-enforcement agencies. One classic Backster experiment involved plant murder. He put two plants next to each other in a room, along with six of his students who each drew from a hat a piece of paper, one of which had instructions for the murder. The people with the five blank pieces of paper left the room with Backster. In the room, the "murderer" ripped one of the plants to shreds. Backster then returned, attached the remaining plant to a polygraph machine, and called the students into the room, one by one. There was no response on the machine to the five innocent students, but when the murderer entered, the pen flew across the paper as the silent "witness" recognized the guilty party.

The implications of Backster's work on plants are staggering enough, but he has also done experiments with other life-forms including eggs, shrimp, and human mouth cells — the implications of which are equally amazing. Backster had to conclude that all nature is essentially unified, not separate.

The planet hums. It emits a low-frequency radio signal, the earth's vibration, which is known as the Shumann resonance. It can be detected coming off trees. Researchers in America were curious to know whether this vibration could be altered with human thought and feeling, and connected an oak tree to a machine described as being not unlike those used to measure brain waves in humans. A group of people circled the tree and, saying a traditional native prayer, sent it love. Apparently, the signal went off the scale. Although the measurements can't really say whether the tree was happy to receive this love or wanted everyone to go away, clearly some form of interaction was taking place.

Plants respond to human thought and to the human energy field, and you can prove it for yourself. In the thought experiment devised by Marcel Vogel, you pick three leaves from the same tree or plant and place them by the side of your bed. Vogel put them on glass, presumably so he could view the underside without touching the leaves, but a sheet of paper will do. Every morning when you wake, concentrate on just two of the leaves, sending them love and pleading with them to live. Imagine them green and healthy looking. Ignore the third leaf. Don't touch any of them for seven days, by which time the leaves you concentrated on should still be looking fresh, while the ignored leaf should be shriveled. Do the experiment when you wake because that's when you're most physically and mentally relaxed. It's absolutely vital to approach this with a pure heart, because plants know what you think. Don't try to fool them because you'll only be fooling yourself. *Expect* the experiment to work.

In the energy experiment devised by Daphne Beall, you put water in a container and energize it by putting both hands around it without touching it. Relax and visualize white-light energy coming out of your hands, into the container. Imagine the water becoming bright white, and do this for ten minutes. Then put a tomato in the water. Get a second container, fill it with water, and put another tomato in it without thinking about it at all. Leave both containers overnight and in the morning take the tomatoes out of the water and place them where they can sit for three weeks without being moved. Put labels nearby so you know which is which, and wait to see what happens!

An energy connects us to plants. In some people it is very obvious, when they transform a neglected piece of earth, as if with fairy dust, into a resplendent garden. We say they have a "green thumb." But everyone has empathy for the glory of nature, natural gardeners or not. There is a magnificence there we can plug into, and do.

It is difficult to see which particular field of study should research the subject of human-plant interaction. It involves the study of light, physics, astrophysics, metaphysics, botany, biology, harmonics, electromagnetics, hydrology, mineralogy, and a dozen other disciplines, plus neurology, philosophy, spirituality, theology, and psychology, to name a few. Perhaps that is why the field is so little researched — we don't know whose academic territory it is! The answer may be, of course, that it is everyone's territory, because there is only one territory, in that we are all part of the connecting whole.

THE SANCTITY OF PLANTS

People have always been spiritual. Indeed, spirituality has been the drive of much, if not most, culture and art throughout time — from Paleolithic cave art created 30,000 years ago to generations of art objects, temples, sculpture, and paintings. People used to so sincerely believe in an afterlife that they made sure their relatives were buried with goods they would need there, including sometimes a fortune in gold jewelry. Today we may question the existence of an afterlife and place any jewelry in our will. Sometimes we don't seem very spiritual at all. Yet even *we* feel it strongly — there must be something else . . .

Where does this spirituality come from? What has made people think there is a life after death and an intelligence that embraces the universe? Some skeptics would say that spirituality is just a tradition of superstition, that people don't have spiritual experiences, they just *think* they do. These people can point to certain evidence. For example, the crystals in granite, being radioactive, cause brain stimulation, including hallucinations, which may explain why granite was used to build the Neolithic *dolmens*, or shelters, and to cover the walls of important rooms like the King's Chamber in the Cheops pyramid in Egypt. Skeptics say people sat in these places and "tripped out" (more or less like an LSD trip) and thought they were having spiritual experiences, but they were only playing with their own minds.

The same skeptical attitude could be taken toward the spiritual use of sound, dance, and plants. Sound in the form of chanting, singing, or the repetition of mantras sets up a vibration that changes brain functioning and can cause a "spaced-out" feeling. Dance can do the same thing. Certain plants are psychoactive — they have an effect on the mind or psyche — and have been used by shamans from South America to Siberia for millennia to facilitate a state of trance and another perception of reality. Some say these activities give a false impression of spirituality, and fear and superstition do the rest.

This is a very limited point of view, for there are many other types of spiritual experiences that don't involve stones, sound, dance, or plants. The basic spiritual experience is love; some people fall in love after knowing each other a very long time, others fall instantly at the sight of a stranger across a crowded room. When a loved one is far away, he or she can be thought about, scanned for in the distant horizon, located, and brought back to our heart through our spirit. We seem connected in a way that defies the laws of place.

Love is spiritual. Also, nature is spiritual, and many people say their strongest feeling of spirituality is experienced among nature, on a mountaintop perhaps, where they are overcome with a strong sense of a beneficent intelligence watching over us all. Many people have spontaneous spiritual experiences, when they suddenly become devout. Others have near-death experiences, see the other side, and come back certain of an afterlife. Many people hear voices — including some of the central characters in the Old Testament — when they're just walking along, not expecting revelation. And people have been bumping into angels for millennia.

It's because the spiritual realm exists that we have this thing called "spirituality." When people use stones, sound, dance, and plants, they are *seeking* to make the connection with something they already know is there. These things are not *the reason for* spirituality but *a means to* spirituality. People want to reconnect, and they feel they need help.

When, in the Bible, Aaron burned incense every morning and evening, it was not to create two little pockets of "spiritual experience" within the day. Aaron felt the spirit all day long. He burned incense to concentrate his mind on the subject . . . and because God had told him to. Likewise, Buddhists don't burn incense to receive the enlightenment of Buddha's words; they already know them and believe them to be the right path to follow in life. Incense is burned to experience the enlightenment directly, to connect with something they know is there.

Certain plants have been chosen as spiritual aids by people living thousands of miles apart, on different continents, in different millennia. Cedar is a case in point. The temple of Solomon in Jerusalem was built with Cedar of Lebanon, and it is possible the Hebrews extracted an oil from the wood. In India, cedar is used to induce trance, while in Native American culture it is said to have the ability to counteract negative forces. Why should these and other peoples choose cedar? Is it because it *smells* good, or because it *does* something in the spiritual realm, or both?

Plant materials have long been used in spiritual practice, and the more fragrant they were, the more spiritual they were considered to be. This may be because fragrance transports. You can be in a place or situation and feel very uncomfortable, with chaos and noise all around you, then close your eyes, inhale a particular fragrance, and bypass it all, reconnecting with the great cosmic whole. It's like a private vehicle silently and instantaneously whisking you away to reconnection; fragrance can be a ticket to the Divine.

ESSENTIAL OILS: THE UNSEEN ENERGIES

In the usual light photographs of the Milky Way, its shape seems obvious: a spiral disk, a basically flat circular shape made up of countless white stars. But when you get on the Internet and look at some of the photographs that have come back from space, you can see that the reality is much more complex. The websites to visit are NASA's Goddard Space Flight Center and the University of Illinois, which display photos of the Milky Way taken using X-ray, infrared, and radio equipment. When the frequency is changed, further levels of reality are exposed. Using computer enhancement and color, different swirls of energy are highlighted, and "bipolar outflows" are revealed as coming out from the center, like two trumpets, perpendicular to the disk of stars. These exciting new pictures illustrate how much more there is to life than what we can see with our eyes.

Life on planet Earth certainly seems more benevolent than on the other planets in the solar system, and more vibrant, but what do people know of its invisible energies? Human energy fields have been recognized in most, if not all, spiritual traditions. Eastern traditions talk of *prana* and *chi*, the energies that are vital to health. In Western terminology, we hear of the aura, or of the etheric body, astral body, mental body, and spiritual body, and a golden web that connects us all. It is likely that we are dealing with several energy fields that interact with one another and our physical selves, and they are said to be the means by which we connect with the Divine.

According to Dr. Valerie Hunt, a physiological scientist and author of *The Infinite Mind: The Science of Human Vibrations*, although the electrons existing in humans and inactive matter are the same, the human field absorbs and throws off energy, while inert matter is passive. In addition to the electrical frequencies

of the muscle, brain, and heart there is "another field of energy, smaller in amplitude and higher in frequency." Apparently this energy is electromagnetic, and
eight to ten times faster than the other electromagnetic energy recorded on the
body's surface. Dr. Hunt has done much research on the human aura, taking
measurements when subjects were in the mountains, near the sea, or after having a swim, a shower, or a barefoot walk on grass, and in special scientific study
environments, such as the Mu and Anechoic rooms at the University of California in Los Angeles. The Mu room, located in the physics department, is an environment in which the electromagnetic energy in air can be altered. When the
electrical aspect of the atmosphere is taken out, subjects in the room find that
they become unaware of the location of their bodies in space, and the aura
becomes scattered. The Anechoic room is designed to take out sound and light, and
thus these sources of electromagnetism, and subjects lose their sense of time and became unable to operate the instruments taken in there for research study.

There are few people in the Western world who have carried out as much
scientific research on the human aura as Dr. Hunt, and she writes in *The Infinite
Mind*:

> The human field looms as primary to life.
> Resonating frequencies are primary physical bonds in nature.
> For every frequency or frequency band, there exists natural or created
> resonators. In other words, a field's frequency pattern at a given time
> is a resonating structure that determines the energy it will absorb or
> by which it will be affected. Theoretically, all frequency vibrations
> exist in the universe (which includes the body) — from sub herzian
> to as high as modern instruments can measure — billions and tril-
> lions of cycles per second. Nonetheless, each material substance, liv-
> ing or inert, mineral or chemical, has its own vibratory signature
> carried in the structure of its field. There are dominant and recessive
> vibrations in each field, giving it character. Field interactions result
> from the strength and pattern of these field vibrations. These consti-
> tute windows, or thoroughfares for transactions.
>
> A sound general principle states that interaction between fields
> occurs when there are compatible harmonic frequencies.

What I believe happens with essential oils is that they are "thoroughfares
for transactions" — they have their own vibrations that connect with the frequencies in the human energy field, causing effects in the physical, emotional,
and spiritual body. Essential oils have different electrical qualities and different

molecular shape and vibration. Interesting though all the data is, it does not explain what one might rather vaguely call "the energy" of a particular essential oil. New methods of recording are required.

With this in mind, I went to see Harry Oldfield, who coauthored with Roger Coghill *The Dark Side of the Brain*, a seminal work on unseen energies when it was published in 1988. Oldfield has invented an energy field imaging system that records the invisible aura of energy around all living things, and I was interested to know what it could reveal about essential oils. According to Oldfield, the images produced show interference patterns with light, as light rays and photons get "interfered with by the subtle energy effects emanating from the object or space point. I say 'space point' because there are atmospheres and places that give off emanations too."

Using this new equipment, which produces moving images on a computer monitor, colorful and dynamic patterns emerge in the air around the end of the smelling strip on which the essential oils are placed. With some, such as jasmine and ginger, the end of the strip appeared bright white, with all the color spectra in that spot. In others, the whole strip appeared energized, while another showed no change. The background is generally green but different essential oils make it explode into color and shape, individual in each case. We saw magenta circles and squares or predominantly purple, orange, turquoise, or blue ones, all actually layers of color much like a rainbow. With *Eucalyptus citriodora* (eucalyptus lemon), a yellow haze appeared, while with frankincense, a sudden rocket of energy flew out from the end of the strip, and with neroli, a blue circle appeared at a distance and started beating like a heart, getting slightly smaller, then larger — a flashing light of life — pulsating seven times before dispersing. The individuality of these essential oil energy patterns is amazing, and the more you see, the more amazing they are!

What we are seeing, Oldfield believes, is the etheric energy in the fabric of space itself, going beyond the molecules themselves, an energy that is in a buffer zone between the physical and higher energies. Some of the essential oils made very little impression and some were very dramatic, and the differences were not related to when, in any particular sequence, the image was taken — first or last or in between. It cannot be said, then, that as the aroma molecules built up in the atmosphere, things got more dramatic. Sometimes, toward the end of a session, there would be an essential oil that showed very little activity. Also, some of the energy fields were very small and remained close to the end of the strip, while others immediately shot out all around and took up much space. In some, the energy field seemed to hover above the smelling strip, then in others it hung below. Some fields seemed to come toward us, some went out, some stayed where they were, while others leaped! The kinetic nature of these events is not captured by the still images reproduced on pages 125–28. In some essential oil recordings, the energy was slow to build up, in others it built up instantaneously.

Discussing the images observed on the computer screen with the other people in the room, I realized that we were using the same vocabulary I use when describing essential oil fragrances in other contexts. Someone would say, "it's round" or "sharp," "sparkly," "heavy," "light," "soft," "dynamic," or that it "has direction."

It was also very interesting to watch the energy field of the essential oil mingle with and affect the aura emanating from a person if the person held the smelling strip or stood nearby. I was reminded of Hunt's phrase "a thoroughfare for transactions." Oldfield's words were emphatic: "They definitely interact in the human energy field, there's no doubt about it." The mystery of the life force of essential oils was looking less mysterious by the minute.

Essential oils are crystalline structures that carry light. They vibrate and cause selective synchronous vibration; they are electromagnetic, as we are ourselves. They are thought to travel through the interstitial fluid, the space between the cells, where the molecules of emotion also travel, as has been shown by psychoimmunologist Candace Pert. Watching the energy of the essential oil molecules was fascinating, and even more so when a human being was included in the image. Then the energy fields from the essential oil and the person gently connected, and we saw an expansion of the human aura. It's no wonder that fragrance has been used since time immemorial to connect people with the Divine, lifting us to finer, higher vibrations, in touch with wider consciousness.

Chapter 2

Using Essential Oils for Spiritual Union

Let the rich fumes of od'rous incense fly,
A grateful savour to the powers on high;
The due libation nor neglect to pay,
When evening closes, or when dawns the day.
— Hesiod, *Works and Days,* i. 334,
eighth century BCE

THE SPIRITUAL CONNECTION could be said to take place within the dynamic energy that permeates the entire universe. It is a space of light and high vibration, and anything used for subtle healing — the reconnection of body to spirit — needs to be in harmony with it.

Essential oils carry the light, and that light potential is activated by positive thought. Even physicists accept that thoughts are a form of energy, saying the human observer has to be included as part of the experiment because that person's thoughts affect the outcome. Thought is part of scientific equations, even though we can't grab a thought and put it under the microscope!

When working with an essential oil for first aid, or for a physical ailment such as rheumatism, although the energetic aspects of the essential oil are important, it is more important to choose an essential oil with the chemical properties essential to do the job required of it. When choosing an essential oil for subtle healing or spiritual connection, however, the chemical constituents are not as important because they are not being required to act on the physical, or chemical, matter of the human body. What is most important is the energy of the essential oil, its vibrational note, which interacts with our own spiritual harmonic note as part of the universal symphony.

Any essential oil distilled from a plant lovingly grown in unsullied soil, under an unpolluted sky, by caring people, and distributed by a company working with integrity and respect, is going to have good energy. Nature vibrates with its own joy of life in which we can share and, indeed, essential oils produced under such favorable conditions appear to have a more beneficial effect on the sick or wounded than those distilled from plants subjected to polluted growing conditions, chemical adulteration, or negative thought forms. When considering using essential oils for subtle healing and spiritual purposes, the energetic aspects of production are equally important.

The first step, then, is to consider the question of supply. Ultimately, after the various mechanical means of purity analysis, there is one judge of aroma, the nose, which is the most direct pathway to the mind and spirit. The way to train a nose is by comparison. Simply open the tester bottles of the various brand-name essential oils and take a whiff. After a while you'll find outlets that carry oils with a purity, clarity, and energy that stand apart from the rest. Take your time though, make it a mission — it's worth the effort. Talk to different suppliers and find out what you can about their sources. Seek, as they say, and you shall find.

THOUGHT, INTENT, AND PURPOSE

Thoughts are very powerful things, and I say "things" because, although they're invisible, they're almost tangible. They seem sometimes to fill the space around a person, so you can know what a person is thinking even when his or her back is turned. Some people even believe thoughts can be impregnated into the fabric of buildings or objects, and that their energy can be felt centuries later. Thoughts certainly travel across space very quickly, and people very often know what someone else is thinking at that instant, no matter where in the world that person happens to be.

When it is *we* who are having the thoughts, they can seem to fill the whole space around us. Sometimes we may feel people can read our thoughts, so obvious are they, so extended from ourselves. They seem to have a power, an energy of their own, even transmitting to other people, sometimes when we wish they wouldn't.

There have now been studies carried out on what is termed "nonlocal quantum phenomena," how one person's thoughts can somehow instigate an effect in another person. Also, research shows that this phenomenon is instantaneous, and it's not affected by distance. It doesn't matter whether the two people are standing right next to each other or on different continents. Although such a concept seems unbelievable, it actually mirrors a phenomenon known by science to occur with subatomic particles. If two subatomic particles that have been in contact with each other are separated, a change made to happen in one also happens, exactly the same and instantaneously, in the other, no matter how distant the particles are from each other. So, if there is a correspondence between human thought and human thought, and between subatomic particle and subatomic particle, why not between humans and essential oils?

As I have written in *The Fragrant Mind*, scientists have established that the chemical composition of the DNA in a moose, the animal, and a spruce, the tree, is essentially identical. Both DNAs are encased in cells, which are structurally the same, and like ours. Moreover, the only chemical difference between chlorophyll in plants and red hemoglobin in human blood is that a magnesium atom in one replaces an iron atom in the other. As Richard Thompson so eloquently puts it in *The Brain, A Neuroscience Primer*, "The similarity of the genetic material in all forms of life that exist in the world today, including bacteria, plants, animals, and people, indicates that all living organisms descended from the same single cell-line." In other words, human beings and plants come from the same familial line and have a relationship. It is that fundamental relationship that can be activated by thought. How poignant it is that all Lakota North American ceremonies end with the words *Mitakuye Oyasin*, meaning, "we are all related," which is a prayer recognizing every living thing. Every person, animal, and plant is part of the same single family.

Of course, essential oils are not living plants, and although someone might be prepared to accept that we can communicate with plants, they might say we can't communicate with essential oils as they are "only" the essence of a plant. I'm reminded of some more work carried out by Cleve Backster, the New York lie-detector expert who proved that plants respond to human thought — he also discovered that if he ground up a leaf he could get the same emotional-electrical results as he did with live plants.

I talked to many people while researching this book and each time the subject of thoughts came up, everyone was emphatic. Yes, they said, the energy of essential oils varies depending on the mind frame of those handling them. Whether I spoke to scientists who take measurements of essential oils, religious leaders, or medicine men, all were in agreement: essential oils have a vibration that is altered by the persons handling them. This fact throws light on a strange (or not so strange) phenomenon: two people using the same species of essential oil can elicit two different responses — one that has the desired effect and one that doesn't. It almost seems as if, in the latter case, the oil has been sapped of its energy; however, it's more likely the case that the light potential in the oil has been switched off and, thankfully, can be rekindled.

The first thing I say to those attending my workshops is that the most important element of handling essential oils is encapsulated in three words — thought, intent, and purpose. *Thought* motivates the action of picking up a particular essential oil, *intent* is about having positive intentions, and *purpose* is what you are trying to achieve; it's the objective.

Basically, we need to stop and think what we are doing and why we are doing it, and apply our head and heart to the process. We want to *see* a good result and use the appropriate essential oils to achieve that result. When using oils with others, smile and *see* the recipient in a completely abundant way: in spirit, mind, and body, their positive qualities enhanced. Don't dwell on any minor irritating aspects the person may have, or impose any private thoughts on the essential oils, such as, "This will calm him down." It is not for us to impress our will or ego on the oils; we merely facilitate the joining of the harmonious energies between them and human beings.

Medical therapists have to do more research than casual aromatherapy users and will be knowledgeable in the therapeutic values of essential oils. They know the potential of any particular species and may invoke that potential as they blend their oils. If a client has an inflammatory condition, as the practitioner rolls the bottle between his or her hands, he or she could think of the anti-inflammatory qualities of the essential oil and ask that energy to come to the aid of the client, not forgetting to kindly thank it. This is energetic blending to a purpose. Sometimes that purpose may be limited; for example, the objective might simply be to turn a sports-damaged knee into a healthy knee. At other times, the purpose may be larger, encompassing spiritual health too, and therapists will want to blend for positivity and happiness.

When using the essential oils at home, for example when taking a bath, make a conscious decision to take the bath in a certain way. Don't let your mind ruminate on whatever thoughts are bothering you at the time. When picking up a bottle of essential oil, think instead of the source of it. If it's sandalwood, think of the thirty-foot-high tree with its inner core, the heartwood that is used in the production of this oil; if it's rose, think of the many-petalled delicate flower. Or take a deep breath and focus your whole mind on a picture you enjoy, a view of nature or something else that brings a smile to your face. Pamper yourself spiritually. Or think of yourself at your most glorious best, as you would wish to be.

PURIFICATION

Nature is remarkably resilient. Think of a little seed lying in the earth, when along comes this massive machine, shaking the ground, moving inexorably toward it, and then it dumps a whole load of cement right on top of the seed to make a path or driveway. You might think, "That's the end of that!" But no, time passes, and a tiny green shoot pops its head through a hairline crack in the hardened concrete, into the light, and grows into a plant. We come along and say, "Look at that, another weed," and pull it out! But more plants grow in its place, and despite everything we do, nature still has that profound drive to live. Essential oils too appear to have that life quality, despite whatever human negativity they get subjected to.

Thoughts are vibratory and essential oils are too. If the vibration of the thought is light, or heavy, the essential oil will respond accordingly. Perhaps even the earth in which the essential oil plant grows is affected by thought. Finding out about the mind-set of the growers, distillers, bottlers, and sellers, however, can be difficult. Going to the fields in which the crop is grown and meeting with the people involved in the process, all the way down the line, is just impossible for most essential oil users. Some aromatherapists do spend a fair amount of their time sourcing, and will drop, or adopt, different suppliers depending on their attitude of mind, be it negative or positive. For the casual user, however, the most practical way to approach the problem is to spend some time clearing the oils. While I do not believe essential oils can do harm energetically, they may not be able to realize their light potential if any negative thought forms have been around them.

Some people invoke the help of God, through prayer, to cleanse their essential oils, or they use the classic decontamination material, salt. Reference is made to it in the Old Testament in 2 Kings 2:21, when Elisha "healed" the springwater at Jericho: "And he said, bring me a new cruse, and put salt therein. And they brought it to him. And he went forth unto the spring of the waters, and cast the salt in there, and said, Thus saith the Lord, I have healed these waters; there shall not be from thence any more death or barren land." At Shinto shrines in Japan, piles of salt are often placed on either side of the Torri arch, to clear negativity from the people entering. In Asia salt is often used to clear away negative energy from people as they enter sacred places. Salt is certainly cleansing, which is why a dentist may tell you to rinse your mouth out with it. But that does not explain why it is so universally used for spiritual decontamination — perhaps because the crystalline structure of salt makes it an attractor. There was a time

What Are Essential Oils?

- Essential oils exist only in *certain parts* of *aromatic plants*, from which they are distilled or otherwise extracted.

- Only *some species* of the aromatic plants are used — there are approximately seven hundred varieties of geraniums, for example, but only ten produce an essential oil that could be used in aromatherapy.

- Only *specific parts* of the essential oil-producing plants are used. Depending on the species, the essential oil might be extracted from the *petals* or *flowering tops, leaves, twigs* or *stems, roots, rhizome, grass, resin, bark, chopped heartwood, fruit* or *seed.*

- The essential oils are found within the plant part in specialized *cells, buds, canals, cavities, ducts, vittae,* and *glands.* Some plants produce their essential oil within "oil hairs," or *glandular trichomes*, extending from the surface of the leaves.

- Usually essential oils are extracted from the relevant part of the plant by *steam distillation.* Essential oils in fruit peel — their "zest" — is extracted by *cold-pressing*, or "cold expression." *Enfleurage*, or *solvent extraction*, is often used with flower petals, as steam distillation is usually too "rough" a process for them.

- The essential oil in petals is often first extracted with enfleurage, then by extraction of the resulting *concrete*, or *pomade*, using natural solvents or CO_2 (carbon dioxide). The end result is called an *absolute* and contains the heavier molecules, as well as the lighter ones that are extracted through the more usual steam distillation. Absolutes contain additional components, in-cluding waxes, color pigments, fatty acids, vitamins, and minerals, making the absolute smell just like the flower itself.

when raw, unrefined sea salt was usually preferred for these purposes, but since the seas are now so polluted, rock salt is probably best.

Making sure the top is shut tightly, put the bottle of essential oil in a glass and cover it with salt. Leave it there for twenty-four hours, then rinse the bottle in springwater and wipe it dry. At this point, if you wish, the bottle can be surrounded by rock crystals, which have themselves been washed in salty springwater and left to dry in the sun. This act should be done with a completely clear mind, as there is absolutely no reason to impose your mind, or even your love and good intentions, on the essential oils at this point. They have their own love and good intent — pure, egoless energy. By carrying out this process, we clear the way for that loving energy to shine through.

HANDLING AND STORAGE

When handling essential oils, you must treat them with respect, for these are living things, and wise healers. At home, keep them where it intuitively feels right, where you feel peaceful and relaxed perhaps, or near a sacred picture or religious symbol, or on a shrine. Many people keep their most precious spiritual articles together, and the essential oils could be kept with them. There are other considerations though. Essential oils don't like light or heat. They should be kept in dark glass bottles and stored away from both artificial and natural light and heat sources. They should also be stored away from sources of radiation and electromagnetism, such as microwaves, computers, radios, CD players, and TVs. It is actually quite difficult to find a place that meets all these requirements in a typical modern home, but with a bit of thought and ingenuity, a suitable place can be found. (Also, there are various devices on the market to counteract these energies.) If your usual sacred area is too light, simply store the essential oils in a box, or make a space for the essential oils in a shaded place, a cabinet for example. You may also choose to put around them some of your other precious and sacred objects — whatever it is that means "sacred" to you. Above all, think of the essential oils as living things that deserve to be treated with reverence because the power of nature, of creation, of light, and of love, is within them.

THE SPIRITUAL CONNECTION

> *And there appeared unto him an angel of the Lord standing on the right side of the altar of incense.*
>
> — Luke 1:11

When you're using essential oils specifically for subtle healing or spiritual enhancement, create a special time to link with the divine energy of the universe. You may plan this, or intuitively decide "this is the time," but whichever it is, approach this time as sacred and special. Mark it out in your mind as qualitatively different from the rest of the day. What you do in that time, in terms of it being a ceremony or ritual of some sort, is not as important as approaching it with the right intention. Empty your mind of negativity, focus on the positive, and recognize the divinity in the energy that pervades all living things. Breathe deeply, slow down, and rest in infinite peace within yourself.

The Heavenly Atmosphere

> ...among the ten thousand rites, the burning of incense has
> the primacy....
>
> — Taoist liturgical text

In the Eastern spiritual traditions of Hinduism, Buddhism, Shinto, and Taoism, the burning of incense is commonplace both during public worship at temples or shrines, and at home. The earliest evidence for the burning of incense in China is dated during the Shang dynasty, which ruled from 1766–1123 BCE. Islam has also been very positive about the use of fragrance, partly because of these words ascribed to the prophet Muhammad: "It has been given to me to love three things in your base world: women, perfume, and prayer, but the apple of my eye is prayer." In Pakistan, Muslims use incense during the ceremonies of circumcision and marriage, and it's burned from the moment a person dies until they are buried.

On the other hand, the Western spiritual traditions of Judaism and Christianity have historically been ambivalent about the religious use of fragrant materials, with different branches of the religions, at different times, being for or against it. The early antipathy to the burning of incense, other than for priestly use, comes from the fact that the religious opposition — goddess worshippers — burned incense in some profusion. In Ezekiel 8:9–14, for example, we hear how "abominations" were taking place in the form of idol worship, with seventy elders, "...every man his censer in his hand; and a thick cloud of incense went up," with women weeping for Tammuz, son and husband of the goddess Ishtar, the "Queen of Heaven." These practices were already ancient at the time, having been imported from Babylon. The early Hebrews were also, of course, familiar with the burning of incense, which was an important aspect of Egyptian spiritual practice. Incense burning became central to Jewish ritual but was controlled by the priests, starting with Moses and Aaron. In Exodus 30:34–37, God ordered Moses to make an incense:

> Take unto thee sweet spices, stacte, and onycha, and galbanum; these sweet spices with pure frankincense: of each shall these be a like weight: And thou shalt make it a perfume, a confection after the art of the apothecary, tempered together, pure and holy: And thou shalt beat some of it very small, and put of it before the testimony in the tabernacle of the congregation, where I will meet with thee: it shall be unto you most holy. And as for the perfume which thou shalt make, ye shall not make to yourselves according to the composition thereof: it shall be unto thee holy for the Lord.

At the Temple in Jerusalem, incense was offered twice a day on the Golden Altar in the Holy of the Sanctuary, and once a year before the Ark of the Covenant in the Holy of Holies on Yom Kippur. The ingredients are listed in the daily siddur, in the early section on offerings: stacte, onycha, galbanum, frankincense, myrrh, cassia, spikenard, saffron, costus, aromatic bark, and cinnamon. Each component of the incense is said to represent part of the community of Israel, and none may be ignored.

In the Christian tradition there has over the millennia been much argument about the use of incense. Adverse associations may have derived in part from the fact that Christians were forced to burn incense before images of Roman emperors as evidence of imperial loyalty, or face execution. By the fifth century it was accepted as a symbol of prayer, but fell into disfavor after the Reformation began in 1517, when Martin Luther nailed to a church door in Wittenberg, Germany, his complaints against the theological establishment. Since then, there has been a great deal of debate, not to say division, among different Christian groups regarding the use of incense, as well as other practices. Today incense is burned in some Anglican churches, and is of course much used in Catholic churches. On the subject of incense, the Reverend Allen Morris says, "There is no attempt to lay down 'recipes' by the Church. The requirement simply is that when burnt, the incense should be able to symbolize the sweetness of Christ's sacrifice, as well as the prayers of the Church rising to the throne of God."

Let my prayer be set forth before Thee as incense.
— Psalm 141:2

Greek Orthodox churches offer up incense every day and at eucharistic and sacramental worship. "On a less formal level," explains Gregorios, Archbishop of Thyateira and Great Britain, "incense is used in the homes in a simple ritual in the morning and at sunset when a member of the household (usually the lady of the house) will offer prayers and incense in front of the family's icons and will then take the incense into each room of the house and also incense the members of the family. Even in those households where the daily offering of incense has less emphasis, the incense will be offered at sunset on Saturday and great festivals — sunset being the beginning of the new day in the Orthodox Church and therefore the beginning of the feast."

There are many types of incense used in homes around the world, such as incense sticks or incense cones, and aromatic plant material placed on burning charcoal. People have had different reasons — secular as well as sacred — for burning fragrance in their environment. It's been used to fumigate against insects and disease, and simply as a perfume, as well as for helping focus during meditation and when offering prayers. Whatever form it comes in, incense obtains its aroma from the aroma molecules of the plant materials from which it is derived — essential oils. When incense is burned, there can be a great deal of smoke, which some people enjoy. For those who don't, essential oils provide another option.

There are many ways of using essential oils in an enclosed environment, but the most usual means is by diffuser. How much essential oil you use depends on the strength of aroma required, the size of the area, and the power of the essential oil(s) being used. Bearing these things in mind, use between six to twelve drops for an average-size room, or more if you wish.

It brings communication with the transcendent.
It purifies mind and body.
It removes uncleanliness.
It keeps you alert.
It can be a companion in the midst of solitude.
In the midst of busy affairs, it brings a moment of peace.
When it is plentiful, one never tires of it.
When there is little, still one is satisfied.
Age does not change its efficacy.
Used everyday, it does no harm.
  — Ten Virtues of Koh (incense),
    compiled in sixteenth-century Japan

Anointing

> *Then the Lord said to Moses, "Take the following fine spices: 500 shekels*
> *of liquid myrrh, half as much (that is, 250 shekels) of fragrant cinnamon,*
> *250 shekels of fragrant cane, 500 shekels of cassia — all according to the*
> *sanctuary shekel — and a hin of olive oil. Make these into a sacred*
> *anointing oil, a fragrant blend, the work of a perfumer. It will be the*
> *sacred anointing oil."*
>
> — Exodus 30:22–25

Anointing was practiced by the ancient Mesopotamians, Egyptians, Syrians, and Persians, as well as by the Hebrews. In Egypt, according to nineteenth-century British perfumer Eugene Rimmel:

> Beside incense, ointment was also offered to the gods, and formed an indispensable part of what was considered a complete oblation. It was placed before the deity in vases of alabaster or other costly material, on which was frequently engraved the name of the god to whom it was offered. Sometimes the king or the priest took out a certain portion, and anointed the statue of the divinity with his little finger. . . . No king could be crowned without being anointed: this was done privately by the priests, who pretended that the ceremony had been performed by a god, in order to convey to the people a more exalted notion of the benefits conferred on their monarchs. [Even mummies were anointed, several times a year, with] sweetly scented oil [which] was poured over their heads and carefully wiped off with a towel carried on the shoulder for the purpose. A priest was generally called in to officiate on these occasions.

Mary Magdalen is sometimes called "the patroness of aromatherapy" because she famously anointed Jesus with a great deal of spikenard in John 12:3–7 and Mark 14:3–8. Jesus sent his disciples out "by two and two" to spread the word, and in Mark 6:13, "they cast out many devils, and anointed with oil many that were sick, and healed them." According to John Halliburton in Dudley and Rowell's *The Oil of Gladness, Anointing in the Christian Tradition*, ". . . there was a good deal of 'do-it-yourself' anointing during [the early Church years]. Phials of oil are passed from holy man to distressed woman, from monkbishop to the terminally sick." Ideally the anointing oil should have been blessed by a bishop, a presbyter, or even a holy man of the desert, but "if absolutely stuck," the oil from a lamp in the church would have to do. Around 405 CE, Pope Innocent I told a bishop that oil consecrated by him "is lawful not for the priests only but for all Christians to use for anointing in their own need or in the need of members of their household."

> *By anointing with the oil, the sick are strengthened and healed, the*
> *catechumens are empowered to resist Satan and to reject sin and evil,*
> *the baptized are sealed with the gifts of the Spirit, and the ministers of the*
> *Church are sanctified in God's service. Through the use of these holy oils*
> *may God's grace be poured forth always upon the Church.*
>
> — Rite for blessing the repository in which
> anointing oils are kept (Catholic Church),
> from the *Book of Blessings,* 1985

In the Christian tradition, the significance of the act of anointing is perhaps best made clear by the words actually used during the holy rites. The following are extracts from the rites of various traditions; the first two extracts are from the consecration of the holy chrism rite and are very similar, although they're from two different churches: the contemporary Anglican and the Reformed Roman. A "+" symbol indicates that a cross is made with the fingers at that point.

> *And so, Father, by the power of your love, bless to our use this mixture of*
> *oil and perfume as a sign and means of your heavenly grace. Pour out*
> *the gifts of your Holy Spirit on those who are anointed with it. Let the*
> *splendor of your holiness shine on the world from every place and thing*
> *signed with this oil.*
>
> — Contemporary Anglican rite, consecration of the holy chrism

> *And so, Father, by the power of your love, make this mixture of oil and*
> *perfume a sign and source + of your blessing.*
> *Pour out the gifts of your Holy Spirit*
> *on our brothers and sisters who will be anointed with it.*
> *Let the splendour of holiness shine on the world from every place and thing*
> *signed with this oil.*
>
> — Reformed Roman rite, consecration of the holy chrism

> *Oh Lord, the creator of all things, by your servant Moses you commanded*
> *the hallowing of ointment made with the mixture of aromatic herbs; we*
> *humbly implore your mercy that you would bestow the grace of your*

Spirit and the fullness of + consecration on this ointment, drawn from a
growing plant. . . . May this mingling of liquids bring to all anointed with
them mercy and safe protection for ever and ever. Amen.

— Pre–Vatican II Roman rite, consecration of the holy chrism

Lord God, you bring healing to the sick through your son, Jesus Christ,
our Lord. May your blessings come upon all who are anointed with this
oil, that they may be freed from pain and illness and be made whole.
Amen.

— Lutheran Church in America and Canada,
prayer for the laying on of hands and anointing the
sick, using olive oil blended with aromatic ingredients

. . . and we pray that we may receive your hallowing, like the chrism
which is poured upon our heads, since the chrism which is poured out is
the Name of your only-begotten Son, Christ our God, through whom the
whole world, visible and invisible, is sweetly scented.

— Byzantine rite, blessing of the holy chrism

The Byzantine chrism is made by combining olive oil with between thirty-eight and fifty-seven aromatic substances, making it one of the most complex synergistic blends ever devised. Different Christian traditions apply holy chrism in differing circumstances, which may include some, or all, of the following: baptism, confirmation, anointing of the deceased, ordination of bishops and priests, consecration and blessing of churches, altars, chalices, and bells. In the Roman Catholic Church, the only requirement is that "some aromatic substance" is added, so there is a fair amount of variation in the constituents. In a private communication, the Reverend Allen Morris says, "it would be proper only for natural fragrances to be used."

Many years ago in the Christian tradition, the use of fragrance by women for cosmetic purposes was sometimes frowned upon because it seemed to indicate a certain frivolity, or because it diverted aromatic resources from their more important spiritual use. Today fragrant materials are much more widely available, especially in synthetic form, but we have forgotten that fragrance is inextricably linked with spiritual practice. Yet what does a woman do when she dabs perfume on her wrist but anoint herself? It seems a profoundly secular act, the height of indulgence, yet it finds echoes in our spiritual past, when people made themselves fragrant to make themselves more acceptable to God.

Although fragrance may have gotten itself a bit of a bad name because of "the fallen woman" syndrome, fragrance was originally used to attract God and the angels, rather than any potential suitor. If we can get past any self-indulgent or even lascivious connotations and understand the spiritual nature of fragrance, then "anointing" in this sense can assume again some of its original purpose and meaning.

In the traditional use of the word *anointing*, oil is always taken as the basic substance used. But if fragrance is the key substance of interest, it can be carried in a water-alcohol solution, as well as by oil. We can make our own spiritual blends of essential oils and use them within an oil-based perfume, or within a water-based spray, like an eau de cologne. The aroma in these circumstances is intended to attract the messengers of heaven and help us become closer to the universal whole, as we carry out our spiritual practice, such as prayer, meditation, or affirmations.

> *Thou lovest righteousness, and hatest wickedness: therefore God, thy God,*
> *hath anointed thee with the oil of gladness above thy fellows.*
> *All thy garments smell of myrrh, and aloes, and cassia, out of the ivory*
> *palaces, whereby they have made thee glad.*
>
> — Psalms 45:7–8

The Sacred Waters

> *And Aaron and his sons thou shalt bring unto the door of the tabernacle*
> *of the congregation, and shalt wash them with water.*
>
> — Exodus 29:4

Water was used by the early Hebrews for cleansing and purifying. Due to a commandment given to Moses by God, in the city of David, Jerusalem, pilgrims went daily in a big procession to the spring, Shilock, the waters of which were said to cleanse and sanctify. The priests had to sanctify their hands and feet with water poured from a golden flask before going to the altar or performing actions of spiritual significance.

Baptism is a Christian sacrament of spiritual rebirth by which the recipient is cleansed of original sin through the symbolic application of water — by immersion, pouring, or sprinkling. Muslims, five times a day, obey these words of the Koran: "When ye prepare for prayer, wash your faces, and your hands (and arms) to the elbows; rub your heads (with water); and (wash) your feet to the ankles. If ye are in a state of ceremonial impurity, bathe your whole body" (Sura 5:7). If water is not available, "clean sand or earth" is to be used instead.

The spiritual nature of water is also seen in India, where the fondest wish of devout Hindus is to bathe in the Ganges River at least once in their lifetime, and to have their ashes scattered on it after death. The river is referred to as *Ganga Ma*, Mother Ganga, and each day countless worshippers can be seen on her shore, chanting prayers and offering flowers.

> *Those who bathe devoutly once in the pure currents of the Ganga, their tribes are protected by Her from hundreds of thousands of dangers. Evils accumulated through generations are destroyed. Just by bathing in the Ganga one gets immediately purified.*
>
> — The Brahmandapurana

The tradition of ritual bathing may go back more than four thousand years on the Indian subcontinent, to the city of Mohenjo-daro in present-day Pakistan. The city was built on a grid system, with each house having a bathroom and toilet, with a clay-pipe drainage system and a "Great Bath" measuring 39 by 23 feet long and 8 feet deep, which was probably used for ritual purification purposes.

Bathing has two meanings from a spiritual point of view. It can denote cleansing before taking part in religious observance, or denote a spiritual transformation, as in baptism. Immersion in water induces a state of relaxation that quite often leads to moments of inspiration, spiritual and otherwise. Water is an incredible substance; it has the ability to replicate and retain in a liquid molecular memory anything that it may have only fleetingly been in contact with, and it can be affected by thought forms projected into it. Dr. David Schweitzer has photographed the effects positive thought forms have upon water. He is one of a current body of scientists who believe that water contains somatids, tiny light bodies, visible light particles that can been seen through powerful electron microscopes. These somatids respond by becoming more active and more energetic when positive thoughts are projected into water, and less active in response to negative emotion. The photographs of water taken from holy or sacred sites show clusters of highly energetic somatids floating in balance, and one can only imagine the powerful effect that prayer may have upon water, and the water in our bodies.

When creating your own sacred waters, run the warm bathwater, then add the essential oil, with the bathroom door closed to ensure the aroma molecules remain in the room. The essential oils are inhaled with the steam and absorbed through the skin by osmosis. As a general rule, use four to six drops of essential oil per bath. This may not seem like a great deal, but just one drop of essential oil will infuse the entire body of water with its aromatic impact. Lie there for at least ten minutes, inhaling the precious fragrance.

Bathrooms sometimes have electrical fans installed in them, often integral to the lighting unit. When you use essential oils for spiritual purposes, the noise and vibration of these fittings may disturb the energy or atmosphere you wish to create, so candlelight would be more appropriate. Some people like total silence as they lie in water, the amniotic fluid of the universe, while others may prefer the sound of gentle music to help them reach the higher realms. Bathing always allows a certain detachment from the stresses of daily life, but with a little extra thought and preparation, and the fragrance of the heavens, the inner core of spirituality can more easily be experienced.

Body Oils

In many Arabian countries, a bride's body is massaged in preparation for the sacred marriage ceremony with oils including orange blossom (neroli), rose, jasmine, and other exquisite perfumes. Her dress is often perfumed, while the bridegroom might be anointed with rose and *oud* (also known as aloes wood). These aromatic extravagances have a very long tradition, and their purpose is not only to purify but to deter the evil spirits, the jinni, from coming to the ceremony.

There is a special sacredness inherent in using essential oils directly on the body. The human being is physical, mental, emotional, and spiritual, and all are precious. As a general rule, to one ounce of carrier oil (thirty milliliters), add between ten to twenty drops of essential oil.

In clinical aromatherapy — the use of essential oils for therapeutic purposes — the choice of carrier oil can be very important to the outcome. This is not necessarily the case with subtle healing. In Western spiritual traditions, two oils stand out as well established and loved — olive oil and almond oil — no doubt because these trees grew in the Holy Land. Olive oil is too heavy for an allover body oil; almond oil is thus a good option when choosing a carrier oil. The words *carrier oil* are interchangeable in aromatherapy with *base oil* and *vegetable oil*.

When making a body oil, put the essential oils into the empty bottle first, and whirl them around to allow them to act synergistically with each other. Only when they are blended, and have become something more than their individual parts, should the carrier oil be added. Put the top on the bottle, turn it upside down a couple of times, then gently roll the bottle between your hands. This action not only ensures complete mixing of the ingredients but energizes the blend.

SPIRITUAL BLENDING

With an extensive knowledge of essential oils, aromatherapists choose which oils to use for a particular client by an informed diagnosis of the client's condition and the decision of how it can best be treated, taking into account the physical, mental, and emotional. The good intent of the therapist or person applying the oils activates the light potential in essential oils.

Just before blending, I look at the client and in that instant know whether another element should be added — the spiritual. As the essential oils are joined together, their colors glow, their voices sing. When they have been synergistically blended, I add the carrier oil and whirl the bottle around in my hands. At that most energetic point, I concentrate with love on the plants from which these essences came, on the sacredness of the fragrance, and the joy they bring. Those thoughts will be transmitted to the blend.

At this point, my mind goes empty, with no thoughts, just a feeling of complete peace and oneness with the oils. I see the energy of the oils and dwell in them for a microsecond, luxuriating in the universal energies of which we are all a part. Then I return to the client and continue treatment in a clinical way, not again thinking about the essential oils, or imposing any thoughts upon them. The blend performs its own mission, transporting the precious molecules, which connect with receptors throughout the body. We are the go-betweens, carrying the catalyst — the essential oils — which will help the mind, body, and spirit to heal itself.

Blending with Prayer and Affirmations

Prayer and affirmations are positive thought patterns, vibrations that can be transmitted to essential oils, especially when blending. Prayer is not something tangible, something you can hold in your hand or measure in a laboratory, although its effects are. Many miraculous healings have been accomplished through prayer. However, when praying for another person, particularly when blending, it is crucial to be quite sure what it is the person wishes for, and in my experience people are very complex and may *think* they want a particular outcome when, in their heart of hearts, they don't. By all means, make a blend of essential oils to give to others, which may help them find peacefulness.

METHODS OF USE

Throughout this book various spiritual practices are described, with suggested methods of use. The following chart is intended as a general guide to the volume of essential oil appropriate for each method. See also Appendix One: Safety Data, pages 317–18.

Any objects used in the process of making a spiritual connection, such as diffusers, bottles, bowls, and candles, should be reserved for that purpose only and set apart from those used in physical healing or environmental fragrancing. The objects should be aesthetically pleasing, and treasured.

ESSENTIAL OIL METHODS OF USE		
METHOD	**AMOUNT OF ESSENTIAL OIL**	**GUIDELINES**
Anointing	1–2 drops in ½ teaspoon of vegetable oil	Dilute the essential oil in an organic vegetable oil. Virgin, cold-pressed olive oil could be used, although you may find the aroma of the olive oil overpowers the aroma of the essential oil. Almond is a good carrier oil to use for anointing.
Baths	1–6 drops	Run the bath, then add the essential oil and swish it around. The door should be shut to ensure the aroma remains in the room. Essential oils can be used in their concentrated forms. For those with sensitive skin, the essential oil can be diluted in a vegetable oil — using 1 drop of essential oil to 1 drop of vegetable oil.
		For salt baths, add 2 drops of essential oil into a teaspoon of salt, mix well, then add to the bath water.
		Some essential oils can cause skin irritation. These include basil, cinnamon, clove, grapefruit, eucalyptus, peppermint, lemon, lime, and thyme. As single oils, the above should be used with caution. In blends, they can sometimes be used in baths, depending on the particular formulation.

ESSENTIAL OIL METHODS OF USE (CONT.)

METHOD	AMOUNT OF ESSENTIAL OIL	GUIDELINES
Body Oils	10–20 drops in 30 ml (1 fluid ounce) vegetable oil	If you're using one essential oil, add it to the carrier oil already in the bottle.
		If you're using a blend of essential oils, put them into the empty bottle first, roll the bottle between your hands, then add the carrier oil and blend again by rolling the bottle between the hands.
		For the uses in this book, it is better to make up small amounts, use them, and remake the body oil as required.
		Label bottles with their ingredients and purpose, adding the date of preparation.
Diffuser	6–12 drops, but more if you wish	*Diffusers used for spiritual practice should be devoted to this purpose alone and not used in any other context.*
		Diffusers, or "burners," have two sections — one for the heat source and one for the water/essential oil. The bowl portion in which the water and oil are put should be nonporous, and thoroughly cleaned between each occasion of use. Put in enough water to allow for evaporation; use already-heated water. Put the essential oil on the water, with the heat source already in place.
Candle	1–4 drops per candle	Light the candle and allow some wax to melt around the wick. Then blow out the candle and add the essential oil to the melted wax. Essential oils are flammable, so ensure none gets on the wick. As the wax starts to solidify, light the candle carefully, preferably using a match rather than a lighter. Aromatic candles can be preprepared for later use.
Hands	1 drop (for both hands), neat or diluted	Put 1 drop of essential oil on the palm of one hand, then rub both palms together. Alternatively, first dilute the drop of essential oil in a small amount of vegetable oil. Holding your hands around your nose and mouth, breathe deeply. If praying, hold your hands in the classic position, palms together and near the face.

ESSENTIAL OIL METHODS OF USE (CONT.)

METHOD	AMOUNT OF ESSENTIAL OIL	GUIDELINES
Water Bowl	3–10 drops	This is a diffusion method. Place a small bowl in the room, away from small children and animals. Put boiling water in it, then add the essential oil. The steam carries the aroma around the room.
Feet Washing	2–4 drops	This is often carried out as a symbolic gesture. Fill a large bowl with warm water. Take a teaspoon of salt, add the essential oil to it, then sprinkle on the water. Gently wipe feet with a linen or cotton cloth.
Hand Washing	1 drop	Put a teaspoon of salt in the palm of one hand, add 1 drop of essential oil to it, then rub the hands together and rub the forearms up to the elbows. Rinse off with running water.
Showers	1–2 drops	Wash as usual. Put the essential oil on a separate washcloth and wipe over yourself, avoiding delicate areas while standing under the running water and breathing deeply through the nose.
Clothing	1–2 drops	Use this method only on clothing that is not valuable to you. Put the neat essential oil on cuffs, where it can be raised to the nose when desired; or on a collar or scarf around the neck, from where the aroma will gently rise to the nose. Viscous and colored essential oils will leave a stain, so avoid oils such as myrrh, benzoin, rose maroc, and chamomile (blue).
Tissue or Hand-kerchief	1–2 drops	Put the essential oil on a tissue or cotton handkerchief, place it in a pocket, and take out and inhale when needed.
Room Sprays	6–10 drops, more if you wish	Use a new plant mister. Put in ½ pint (250 ml) of warm water, with ¼ teaspoon of salt and the essential oils, and shake well. Spray high into the air, avoiding polished wood surfaces and materials that could be damaged by either water or essential oil.

	ESSENTIAL OIL METHODS OF USE (CONT.)	
METHOD	**AMOUNT OF ESSENTIAL OIL**	**GUIDELINES**
Fire	1 drop per log or piece of wood	Preprepare wood for the fire by putting the essential oil on each log or piece of wood. Leave for at least one hour before putting on the fire. Take care, as essential oils are flammable.
Incense	3–5 drops	Essential oils can be added to fragrant twigs, incense cones, incense sticks, or granule-type incense that is placed on charcoal. Leave to dry before use, as essential oils are flammable.
Vision Pillows	1–2 drops	Use essential oils on pillows to encourage sweet dreams or visions. Put the essential oil on a corner, where it will not come in contact with the eyes, or on a cotton ball, which can be tucked inside the pillowcase.
Perfume	Dilute the essential oil with jojoba oil (50/50)	Use a small amount, as you would a perfume. Avoid getting it on clothing.
Sweat Lodges	5–10 drops	Mix the essential oil with the water that is to be placed on the hot stones.
Smudge Sticks	1–4 drops, depending on the size of smudge stick	Smudge sticks are bunches of dried, aromatic plant material, usually associated with Native American culture. Essential oils can be added to the plant material. Alternatively, put the essential oil on a smelling strip or stick.

Carrier Oils

Most essential oils in their pure state are too highly concentrated to be used directly on the skin, so they are first diluted in a carrier oil. For example, one drop of essential oil may be all you need to use. That amount will not spread very far by itself, but diluted in a base oil it will cover quite a large area. Good carrier oils are almond oil, apricot kernel oil, grapeseed oil, and macadamia oil. Almond oil is easily obtained, has therapeutic qualities of its own, and can be used by almost everyone. Although olive oil has a venerable position in the Bible, it is too heavy for allover body use.

There is a wide range of carrier oils available, and the words to look for on the bottle, which indicate quality, are *organic*, *cold-pressed*, and *virgin*. Organic denotes that the plant material was not grown using biocides: that is, pesticides, herbicides, or fungicides made using synthetic chemicals or petrochemicals. Cold-pressed indicates that the oil has not been through a heating process to extract the oil from the seed or other source material. Virgin signifies that the oil came from the first pressing of the oil material.

BLENDING ESSENTIAL OILS WITH CARRIER/BASE OILS FOR THE BODY: QUANTITIES TO USE				
Number of drops of essential oil to use	Blend the number of essential oil drops on the left into the volume of base oil on the right, which is either in milliliters or spoonfuls			
Essential Oil	*Vegetable Oil*			
MIN. TO MAX. DROPS	MILLILITERS	TEASPOONS	DESSERT SPOONS	TABLESPOONS
½–1	1	1	–	–
1–5	5	1	1	1
2–10	10	2	1	1
3–15	15	3	1	1
4–20	20	4	2	1
5–25	25	5	2	1
6–30	30	6	3	2

Special Care

Pregnant or Lactating Women: Women who are pregnant or breast-feeding need to be aware that there are certain essential oils that should not be applied to the body during pregnancy or lactation, and these are listed below. In all other methods, women in this condition should use the minimum quantity of essential oil recommended in any particular section. (The oils listed here are in addition to those that should not be used by anyone, which are listed in Appendix One: Safety Data, page 317.)

Aniseed	Clove	Oregano
Basil	Cumin	Parsley Seed
Bay	Fennel	Peppermint
Birch	Hops	Pimento Berry
Black Pepper	Hyssop	Rosemary
Cedarwood	Juniper	Sage
Cinnamon	Mace	Spikenard
Cistus	Marjoram	Tarragon
Clary Sage	Myrrh	Thyme
	Nutmeg	Valerian

People on medication: Use half the recommended dosages. For example, if directions state, "Use four to ten drops," use between two and five drops.

People using homeopathy: Some homeopathic doctors consider essential oils and other strong smells to negate the effects of homeopathic treatments.

Tranquilizer addiction: Use half the recommended dosages. For example, if directions state, "Use four to ten drops," use between two and five drops.

Substance addiction: Use half the recommended dosages. For example, if directions state, "Use four to ten drops," use between two and five drops.

Alcohol addiction: Use half the recommended dosages. For example, if directions state, "Use four to ten drops," use between two and five drops.

Chapter 3

Prayer and Meditation

Seek and you shall find; knock and the door will be opened to you.
— Matthew 7:7

HUMAN BEINGS HAVE ALWAYS YEARNED to contact infinite consciousness; they reach out and find. The two universal ways this can be done is through prayer and meditation. Prayer is very proactive, in that we have something specific on our minds and ask for it in faith. We ask for healing, help in finding love or a job. We entreat with emotion. We ask for blessing and give thanks. Meditation, on the other hand, is passive. We empty our minds, stop thinking about health, love, and our jobs, and go deep within. We try to go beyond the cluttered mind, past the senses, the intellect, the creative impulse, and past even the spiritual layer of ourselves, to complete merger in cosmic consciousness.

It's said that prayer is our way of contacting God, and meditation is the means by which we get the reply. But prayer also gives the reply; it is a two-way channel of communication. Meditation certainly offers a reply, in that answers to unposed questions might come upon a person, but it is also a way of reaching the light and wisdom of God. Both are about communication with the divinity, although prayer reaches out, and meditation, in. Prayer reaches out in supplication and humility, recognizing our connection with the Divine and our familial relationship, saying, "Our Father, who art in heaven . . ." Meditation also recognizes a familial relationship between the original creative force that gave rise to the vibrations of the universe, now manifest in countless physical forms, including us. The connectedness of things beyond our immediate life is at the root of both prayer and meditation, and that which we yearn for. The warmth of connection enfolds us like a mother's arms, giving reassurance and comfort, and the strength to go on.

Fragrance has accompanied many prayers to heaven. It provides the heavenly scent that can act as the focus for meditation and as an avenue, a pathway, a conduit, or a rocket to the stars. Fragrance opens the consciousness, relaxes the mind and body, and puts us in another space — one where we are open and receptive to spiritual exploration.

PRAYER

A woman who did not believe in God went into labor. A couple of hours later she was oblivious to everything in the delivery room, unaware of how many people were there or what was going on. She was in another, very deep place, and started repeating the words, "Oh God, oh Jesus." She prayed for help when it was most needed, like many people, turning to prayer in times of great need, almost unwittingly. Other people have faith every day. They consciously believe in something or some One, and when they pray, they have a direction in which to focus their thoughts. Faith is like love: it's either in you or not, to a varying degree, and sometimes it is hidden deep within.

Someone might ask, "How can you believe in a God? Who has ever seen Him?" Yet this same person might believe there are "wormholes" in space, because scientists have calculated so, although nobody has ever seen a wormhole either. Some people acquired faith in childhood, because it was all around them and they felt it too. Some find faith suddenly, as it hits them like a thunderbolt, while others feel a shimmer of faith within them and seek to expand the light.

Prayer is a way of contacting and tapping into higher spiritual knowledge, a connection to higher realms, the means by which we connect to the heavens and God. It's an interface between us and the universe, a way in which the small voice may be heard. We give thanks, or ask for miracles. People reach for the intergalactic telephone every time grace is said at the dinner table — either alone on a private line, or with the family making a conference call. Jesus said we should ask for our daily bread, ask forgiveness for our trespasses, and that we be delivered from evil. And many people still do this: ask for a raise at work, for forgiveness for doing what they know to be wrong, and for protection from the hard world outside. Throughout the millennia, all over the world people have sought help, and some have had their prayers answered. In 1997, *Newsweek* magazine published the results of its prayer survey: 87 percent said God answered their prayers.

In scientific experiments involving humans, skeptics can always say that psychosomatic influences are involved — that the human mind imagines things. This can't be said with plants. It is, then, interesting to know that when plants are prayed for — to grow healthy and lush — they respond positively. Rev. Franklin Loehr, author of *The Power of Prayer on Plants*, carried out 100,000 measurements on 27,000 seedlings, resulting from 700 experiments involving 150 praying people. He concluded that plants that had been prayed for, in relation to the control groups, germinated earlier, grew faster and with more vigor, had a better chance of survival, and had greater resistance to insects.

Since the 1960s there have been around 300 scientific trials exploring the possibility that the human mind can affect living matter at a distance. In 1990 Daniel Benor reviewed 131 trial reports in a paper entitled *Survey of Spiritual Healing Research*. The subjects influenced during the trials included humans, mice, plants, red blood cells, fungi/yeast, enzymes, and bacteria. In 56 cases, positive results of the trials were found to have less than 1 chance in 100 of being due to chance, and in an additional 21 cases the chance was between 2 and 5 in 100. In scientific terms these are significant results, showing that the mind can influence living matter.

How this may come about is, of course, the big question. In prayer, we invoke change by using thought, sometimes accompanied by the sound of our voice. Both thought and thought/sound go out into the ether, carrying their vibrational patterns, and causing change. The emotion behind the thought gives an additional charge to the vibrational pattern. Perhaps all this can be picked up or received by higher beings, who operate outside our usual visual range and physical realm. These celestial messengers may be angels or guardian spirits, who transmit — by ever finer vibrations — to the next realm and beyond, until our thought makes contact with the universal whole, or God. Perhaps God hears our tiny voice in the ether, with no messengers in between. These things remain a mystery.

Science is equally mysterious. After years of experiments exploring notions around (John Stewart) Bell's theorem, which states that reality is nonlocal, physicists now claim that subatomic particles that were once in contact always remain in contact, even if on opposite sides of the universe, or planet. This can be measured because a change in one such particle elicits the same change in the other, whatever the distance, and instantaneously. If we all came from the same atomic source, even a *very* long time ago, we are all related, and related to the ultimate source, which some call "God." Some subatomic molecules are now more related to others, but ultimately, we all came from the same place. Is it not then possible to conceive that — to varying degrees — all molecules of the universe have this bizarre (but natural) ability to communicate instantaneously with each other, and act upon each other?

The word *pray* is derived from the late Latin word *precare*, "to entreat." This word carries a humble connotation, with supplication, and in times of great need we may appeal to God in some desperation. More usually, though, prayer is like talking to a good friend on the telephone, a reassuring, happy time. The difference is that unlike any human friend, the friend at the end of the universal telephone line knows everything about us, and all our secrets, so there's no point in trying to hide anything. We can be totally honest.

Prayers are not always answered. Earthquakes, tidal waves, tornadoes, and hurricanes sweep the planet and cause loss of life and destruction, despite prayers. People become ill and even die, although they lead exemplary lives and are needed here on earth. These facts have deeply disturbed people and given rise to much spiritual despair. Like many others, I have explored these questions through various spiritual traditions, some of which explain it by karmic law and reincarnation, others by divine retribution and "the sins of the fathers." Others believe God does not intercede in the lives of individual people, while some think in terms of "life's lessons" or "purpose served."

The natural events are fairly easy to understand, as the planet — upon which we all depend — must be allowed to move and breathe at its own pace. It takes precedence over us. As for unwell people, that is the mystery — not surprisingly, as we can't see the whole picture. If we knew *everything*, perhaps even their suffering would make sense. Plus a good deal of suffering is brought upon oneself, or is the result of other human beings acting on us — "it's all man's fault," and God punishes us collectively. All this is very difficult, but if nothing else, it makes us question things, including what we do to ourselves, to other people, and to the planet. This dynamic may work like this: Say there is a cluster of child leukemia cases in a particular location. It is tragic and society questions the cause. A nearby nuclear plant is thought to be the source of contamination and the plant is closed. In the very long term the planet will benefit, as there will be less radioactive waste dumped on and in it. In the short term, the children suffer; in the long term, the planet lives. Although the children and their parents might think they are suffering alone, we are thinking of them, and they are providing the fuel of determination that drives many an antipollution campaign. This is just an example of cause and effect, the parameters of which are difficult for individual sufferers to see. There are many other such examples, and examples of suffering that seem totally needless. But there may be factors in the equation we cannot guess at, even maybe that which we tell our children when people die: "The angels needed them."

Given that not all questions or prayers can be answered, prayer still offers many benefits. It provides peace and spiritual upliftment, offers hope for good health and help in all forms, allows us a chance to express thanks for our blessings and the space to question ourselves or our situations, and provides the courage to help us change. In prayer, we arrive at a quiet place, a place of spirit. This place is in our hearts, there when we need it, and it has been a sanctuary for many people on this earth who have suffered greatly, as hostages or those under torture, for example, who say that being able to escape to that place of prayer was the thing that pulled them through.

It's easier to contact the higher vibrational beings when we have the atmosphere, the peace, and relaxation, when everyday thoughts don't crowd our minds and we can be still, for it is in the stillness that God's love and peace can be felt. And, perhaps, in that stillness we can hear the voice.

"Dear God..."

What are the thoughts and entreaties that fill the space between God and us? In the *Newsweek* survey, 73 percent thought prayers asking for help in finding a job were answered. With the emphasis placed today on monetary success, it's hard to believe that the space between us and the diety isn't clogged with millions of prayers asking to win the lottery, but 36 percent of the respondents said they never pray for financial success. Probably they realize those thoughts have little importance in the spiritual world, whereas words like "Show me a way to transcend my present situation" have.

In prayer, we can commune with the universe, ask questions, and tell of our sorrows, our joys, the good things, the funny things. What we truly wish to pray for often emerges in the process of prayer itself. We might give thanks, say "please," or ask for guidance to be shown a better way of doing things, a better way of understanding, a way to feel more forgiving, or a way to be able to feel more love, compassion, and empathy. And in making the request, we have already taken the first steps toward feeling these things.

Taking the Pathway to Heaven

In the Christian tradition, prayer often takes place on the knees, with hands together. Native Americans stand looking upward, with their hands outstretched and facing the sky, while Muslims put their heads to the ground. Beyond the basic physical position adopted, however, few are taught in any detail how to pray. We may even be given the wrong information. I was taught, for example, to pray only for others, not myself. It took me years, and a certain amount of guilt, to get beyond this notion and accept that it was okay to pray for myself.

In the process of praying for ourselves, we often learn what it is we truly want, which may be very different from what we *think* we want or what we tell other people we want. So imagine this, people praying for other people, without being in a position to know what they really want. Indeed, we may not be getting what we need because someone else is praying for the opposite!

I often hear accounts of people who, so distressed at the thought of losing a partner, sit at the deathbed, sometimes for days, willing that person to live. The partner may themself be praying to die in peace, without having to worry about the other taking it so badly. Any such cross-purpose of wills can take many forms, including praying for people who don't actually want to get better. Doctors and healers of all kinds are very familiar with this syndrome, when someone puts up an often subconscious barrier to healing. In these cases, it may be better to pray that the person is led to understand why they do not really want to get better.

Prayers are often tainted with ulterior motives. I've heard people say they want a loved one to live forever, or at least until they themselves die, and they pray for that, although the loved one may be in great pain and would prefer to die right away. I recall one woman saying to me that she didn't want her husband to get well enough to come out of the hospital until she'd had a chance to redecorate the bedroom; and another who wanted her partner to get better extra quickly so he'd be home in time for her birthday. Better perhaps to pray that the person being prayed for gets his or her own prayers answered!

Many people find it easier to communicate with a messenger of God, an angel perhaps, because the Divine or the infinite consciousness is so awesome. Fair enough, but just make sure you don't pray *to* the angel and make an idol out of it. Give the message to the messenger, *as* a message.

Many people find it awkward or embarrassing to pray, and for them written prayers may provide a good solution. The same sacred place in the mind, as used in thought or spoken prayer, can be used when writing down what it is you want to say — in a relaxed way, aware of the divinity that permeates all existence. Some put their written prayer in a special place, or create a prayer box, or burn the prayer and watch the smoke ascend to heaven. In the Shinto religion, prayers are written on little blocks of fragrant cypress wood, which are kept at the temple for that purpose, and then thrown in the fire. Essential oils can be used in a similar way, fragrancing the paper kept in a box or elsewhere and being an olfactory reminder of the prayer in that place, or essential oils can be put on the paper prayer before it's burned. In ancient times fragrant materials were routinely burned at the time of prayer and, indeed, the origin of the word *perfume* is the Latin *per fumin*, which means "by smoke." Alternatively, prayers can be written on a banner, as in Tibet, and hung outside to blow in the wind. These writing methods may also appeal to people who express themselves better on paper than they do verbally.

Some people speak their prayers out loud, others say them silently in their minds, but why not sing your prayer? There is a whole science to sound, the spiritual use of which includes chanting and the repetition of mantras, as well as song. Sound sets up frequencies in your whole being, as well as in the space that connects you to the Divine. Singing is a very open activity — it opens the heart, allows and even demands a flow — which tends to make things spontaneous and honest. Openness and flow help the prayer reach its destination.

Prayer can take place anywhere — on the top of a mountain or at the supermarket checkout. You see those people on the street? Some of them are walking along silently praying. People pray on buses, trains, or planes, or while walking through a forest. Often, when out and about, the desire to pray comes upon us, and when a prayer is spontaneous it comes from a place deep inside. It is heartfelt and well received. Feel how the prayer rises from the depths of your being and escapes, riding on your emotion, into that space where it can be heard.

Prayer is quite often presented as a bargain: If this prayer is answered, I'll pray every day, go to church or to the temple every week, help out at the hospital, or be a better person. Such bargains are seldom kept. They may work for a while but then things drift back to normal. The cosmic consciousness that can see our past, present, and future knows that.

Suffering has played a part in certain branches of the Hindu, Muslim, and Christian traditions, with people wearing hair shirts and beating themselves with whips. On a less dramatic scale, many people say to themselves, "If I *really* suffer, surely God will answer my prayers." God may not want you to suffer. Try to reach for the light in the faith that things will get better, secure in the knowledge that God will help you if you help yourself.

There's no point in praying for world peace if you constantly argue at home or at work. Better to pray for peace in your own environment and for understanding as to why disagreements arise.

People who have never prayed, or have not prayed for a long time, may find themselves uncertain as to whether they're supposed to kneel, sit, or stand, turn on the lamp or light a candle, put on some music or sit in silence. Regular prayer eventually irons out these questions, and a personal routine is found, one that has evolved naturally and you feel comfortable with. The prayer can start out extremely simply, and then just be repeated, until you feel you want to add another, or a different, element. As time goes on the whole process will become more refined.

In my practice I've often heard people say they're worried they won't be able to kneel in church because of their arthritic knees. I say, "Really, I'm sure God won't mind," but they worry still, so indoctrinated are they in the "right" way of doing things. It's sad we should think there is so little understanding in heaven. Surely, God is accepting enough not to worry about a knee that is not flexible. All our prayers will be heard if they are genuinely said.

As we ask to be forgiven, so too we can forgive, and accept, and contribute to universal forgiveness. We must be honest though, to ourselves as well as to God. This may be hard to start with, but from shy and hesitant beginnings, eventually the whole truth will come out, and we'll feel better for it.

Prayer should not be a duty but something truly meant. We could read from a standard religious text, or turn to a beautiful poem or a passage from a book that strikes a spiritual resonance in us. It's important to be relaxed in prayer, and that is easier when we're genuine and follow our genuine needs. Prayer has always been a wonderful aspect of human experience, and there seems to be a space reserved in our minds and hearts for it. From this inner-most space we travel along a pathway of light, free from mental clutter and genetic memory, past the anguish and the fear, to that place of infinite peace that awaits us like a shelter in a storm or, on a good day, the most brilliant sun. What gets us there most surely is love, the most powerful voice or force in the universe. If the message is to get through, it needs love behind it. God is love, and love is what God hears.

Blocks in the Flow

There are many people who would like to pray, and even think they *ought* to pray, but somehow feel they can't. There are others who dare not or simply do not ask for what they seek because they have mental and emotional blocks that interrupt the flow between them and the deity, causing eddies of distortion in the vibrational pattern their prayers would otherwise create. There are many issues in prayer, and it can take time to sort them out. In the meantime, simply ask that a highway of communication between you and the divinity be established, and that you'll find the strength to remove some of the blocks that may stand in your way.

Fear

We live in a fear-based society, where everything hangs on threats and the fear of them being carried out. We live in fear of losing our jobs, of not being able to pay the bills, of getting ill. Even the idea of prayer can raise its own form of fear — the fear we won't do it correctly. There's also the fear of being hurt in love again. So although we may pray for true love, there may be an emotional blockage to giving or receiving love. In this case, pray to help remove the fear of being hurt.

ESSENTIAL OILS TO HELP DISSIPATE FEAR			
Frankincense	Cypress	Rose Maroc	Cedarwood
Chamomile Roman	Sandalwood	Basil	Coriander
Ginger	Bergamot	Cinnamon	

Guilt

Guilt is one of the most widely used weapons of manipulation, applied most often in the religious, family, or personal relationship areas of human life. Some people carry guilt because they feel they don't pray enough, or because their religious organization makes them feel they should attend *every* service or festival, happily and joyfully. Today there is lot of guilt surrounding issues of health: we're made to feel we caused our own illness by eating the wrong food or having the wrong attitude. Whatever the root cause or causes of guilt, when we do pray that guilt may accompany our thoughts.

The other side of guilt is forgiveness, and this is one of the main things people ask for in prayer: "Forgive us our trespasses." We are also told to ask for help in forgiving people who have hurt us, but what about forgiving *ourselves*? If we can forgive ourselves and dissipate the guilt, it clears and purifies the paths of connection to the higher realms.

ESSENTIAL OILS TO HELP DISSIPATE GUILT			
Linden Blossom	Jasmine	Pine	Rose Otto
Juniper	Clary Sage	Benzoin	Clove

Unworthiness

If we're told enough times that we are unworthy, we may end up believing it. This causes many problems, but in terms of prayer, we may pray for an improvement in circumstances while at the same time believing we don't deserve it. If the unworthiness is indoctrinated into a person during childhood, it is quite often the case that he or she gravitates toward the circumstances and people that reinforce that idea. However, later in life many people realize what they have been subjected to and shake off the shackles of unworthiness.

Wherever you may be in terms of unworthiness, remember, nobody is so unworthy they cannot pray and accept what is given. If you feel unworthy, pray that help may be given to you as you try to find a sense of worth.

ESSENTIAL OILS TO HELP DISSIPATE FEELINGS OF UNWORTHINESS			
Frankincense	Sandalwood	Neroli	Cedarwood
Rose Maroc	Ylang Ylang	Clove	
Cardamom	Mandarin	Geranium	

Receiving and Accepting

Another block to the flow of prayer is the inability or unwillingness to receive. Some find it difficult to receive or accept compliments, gifts, or good wishes without immediately feeling the need to give the same in return. Or they may find it difficult to accept advice or wise comments. But in prayer, we must be receptive to receive the blessings and answers from above. Often these heavenly messages come fleetingly, softly, and gently. They glide into the subconscious, and then into the conscious, so subtly and lightly that if we are not open to receive, we might not recognize that they have come to us, or we may even ignore them.

ESSENTIAL OILS TO HELP US RECEIVE LOVE		
Rose Otto	Neroli	Chamomile Roman
Lavender	Mandarin	Orange

Giving and Letting Go

When you give in prayer — be it words, secrets, supplication, adoration, praise, or gifts — do not expect something in return. You may be blessed, you may not. But giving in expectation is bribery and bargain, which has no place in the spiritual realm. Give generously, because you want to.

True prayer also involves letting go of that part of ourselves that ties us to the cruder vibrations and prevents us from contacting our higher self, or spirit, the voice of which is more easily heard in heaven. It is better to give up preconceived ideas, because spirituality is an adventure into vast, unexplored territory, and individual to each person. There is no need to give up your conscious *self*, only to offer your whole and higher self.

ESSENTIAL OILS TO FACILITATE LETTING GO			
Pine	Tuberose	Carnation	Lemon
Coriander	Frankincense	Cypress	Cardamom
Myrtle	Juniper		

Creating Your Spiritual Haven

Among the wealthy in ancient Egypt, the preparation for prayer was very thorough. They had a separate room, which was sprayed with a scent very much like almond blossom, presumably one of the older varieties. Before prayers, they bathed and put on white raiments. Likewise, all over the ancient world, people put a special place aside for that which dominated their lives — the spiritual. There is nothing new in creating a spiritual haven and, indeed, all over the world people still do it today. Even the poorest Indian home has a space where an image of Siva or Krishna, or one of the other many faces of the deity, watches over the whole household, in front of which there's a small shrine for burning incense and saying prayers. No Catholic home is complete without a picture of Jesus or the Virgin Mary, in front of which eyes will be closed, hands put together, and prayers said. All over Asia, countless images of Buddha adorn quiet, fragrant prayer corners. At any one moment in time, literally millions of people all over the world will be in the midst of deep prayer in their own homes.

We create a spiritual haven so we can have a special place to focus on the spiritual, and contact the higher realms. It's a place we will come back to time and time again, perhaps for different reasons. We may go there to seek peace, focus our minds, clear our thoughts, or just be. And it is there where we can open our hearts to the love in the universe that waits to receive us. Aim to create a peaceful, restful place where the mind, body, and soul can concentrate on themselves, and be whole. It will be a place where you can draw the angelic beings close and make your connection to the universe, and God.

Most of us do not have the luxury of having a whole room to spare, but we can usually find a corner somewhere. That may be in the living room, the bedroom, the study, even the hall. *Where* it is, is less important than what's in it — especially love. It is love in a house or place that makes it a lovely space to be in. The most beautifully decorated palace is not beautiful if no love is generated there. It is the atmosphere of love that makes the haven spiritual. The vibration of love, clear of negativity, carries prayer to its destination.

If you have never created a prayer space before, start by cleaning the area, and whole room, thoroughly. If it is in a family room, do it when you are alone. Clean everything, even inside closets and cabinets, and have every ornament sparkle. While you do this, focus your mind on the Divine, and imagine beautiful colored lights, all the colors in white light, streaming into the room. If you like, play your favorite uplifting music, something that fills you with optimism and joy.

If you wish, the cleansing can be done with salt, which has long been used as a spiritual purifier. First, open the windows and say a small prayer. Then put the salt around the room before you vacuum, using a little in all the corners, including those in wall cabinets, starting away from the window and moving toward it. This dispels any uncomfortable feelings that may have adhered to the fabric of the room.

When your sacred haven area is clean, think of what you will put in it. Start with a small table, and if you don't have one, use a solid box. Cover it perhaps with a beautiful clean cloth, then arrange some favorite or precious things on it. What these objects are is an entirely personal matter. They might include a gift from a friend, or a drawing by a child that makes love rise in your heart.

Many people put a sacred or beautiful picture at the back, standing up on the table or attached to the wall. A plant brings life to the scene and will respond to the love you give in your prayers. Flowers are gifts that brighten our lives and are a joy to focus on as we contemplate the beauty of creation. Put them in your best vase, and change the water regularly to keep them happy. Everyone has their own favorite flowers. For some it is the tall white lily; for others, the tiny white daisy that dots our lawns. In each bloom, we can see the spirit of the flower helping to create the atmosphere of peace.

Add anything else that means something to you spiritually. That may be a crystal, a stone, or a bunch of herbs. It may be a few small treasures gathered over the years. Candles are often lit in spiritual places, perhaps because they represent the spirit within us and signify change and transformation. We can focus on that light, and see the aura glow. Many cultures speak of a purple flame, the flame within. Finally, put your diffuser on the table, adding a tiny amount of salt to the water in the bowl.

Now sit back for a moment and feel the peace *you* have created. Light the candle, representing fire and spirit, which will symbolically burn your words and send them up to heaven, and light the candle under the diffuser, representing light and soul, which will release the fragrance molecules and send them to their source. Then drop between three to ten drops of essential oil into the bowl of the diffuser. Sit quietly just looking and sensing the peace and restfulness, then ask for blessings on your spiritual haven.

The most important thing about maintaining your spiritual haven is to keep negative energies away. Try not to have arguments in this area, or a telephone nearby. As every person you have contact with influences you to some extent, and leaves something of their spiritual frequency in your subconscious mind, so a place is subtly changed by the people who come into contact with it, especially you.

Heaven Scent

As far as we can tell, people have always used fragrance to contact the spiritual realms. This is because fragrance performs many roles. It helps the mind to focus and concentrate. It also relaxes the mind and body, and opens the heart so it can receive. More than this, though, it creates a link between the conscious and subconscious mind, allowing a chain of events to come forth. It expands the space between thoughts, the space that leads to the oneness of the universe.

Which essential oils you use for spiritual purposes is very much up to you.

This is a personal journey, and a matter of personal choice. Each fragrance suggested is only that, a suggestion. For each person a fragrance will resonate at a different tone and rate. Find which oils or blends resonate with you and keep those fragrances close to your heart.

Although you may have favorite perfumes or fragrances that you use in your daily life, they are not the ones to use now. For spiritual purposes, choose something new and different, something that can lift you from your ordinary existence into the realm of the spiritual. The fragrance we use now is ultimately chosen to assist in prayer. The following are some of the fragrances that have been used in spiritual practice and ceremony, by various cultures around the world.

FRAGRANCES USED IN SPIRITUAL PRACTICES AROUND THE WORLD
Trees
Cedarwood, Cypress, Ho-wood, Juniper, Pine, Rosewood, Sandalwood, Silver Fir, Spruce
Herbs
Basil, Cistus, Hyssop, Marjoram, Myrtle, Rosemary, Sage
Resins
Balsam, Balsam de Peru, Benzoin, Frankincense, Galbanum, Myrrh, Styrax
Flowers
Carnation, Chamomile, Hasmine, Hyacinth, Narcissus, Nerolim, Rose, Tuberose
Roots
Ginger, Spikenard, Vetiver
Spices
Black Pepper, Cinnamon, Clove, Nutmeg
Fruits
Juniper Berry, Lemon, Orange, Yuzu

For those who like to walk through woods, the essential oils extracted from trees are very helpful. There are throughout the whole world many species of pine, cedarwood, and cypress, and these three are universally used in spiritual practice. If you are Japanese you may feel a particular resonance with hinoki pine, which is indigenous to Japan, while if you are North American, the Virginia pine may strike a chord with you. People from Europe may prefer the fragrance of Scotch pine, and those from India, sandalwood.

Resins have long been used in the making of incense, all over the world. The material lends itself to the purpose particularly well, but there has also been a symbolic association, in that resins seep from wounds in trees, as blood saps from us. In ancient Egypt, nuggets of resin were known as "the sweat of the gods," and collected in reverence.

Resins, including balsam, feature strongly in biblical fragrance. Frankincense and myrrh are still burned regularly in many churches and are particularly evocative of the Christian tradition. Benzoin, on the other hand, is more commonly used in spiritual practice in Asia, for example in India, Malaysia, and Java. In general, the fragrances of the resins are not as familiar as, say, the aromas of the herbs. To discern, then, whether they appeal to your higher self, explore them aromatically. The resins and root essential oils can be very pungent and are therefore usually used in small quantities.

The fragrances of flowers are particularly effective when connecting with the angelic realms. And don't forget the fruits, which have wonderful focusing and concentrating properties, individually or in blends.

When essential oils are used in spiritual practice, especially in diffusers, there is a great deal of choice. If we have no heavy thoughts, the lighter essential oils are generally more appropriate than the heavy types. In cases where a person is down and heavy of heart, although you might think a light essential oil is better for the job of upliftment, the headier oils seem to be better suited to do the job, at least to start with.

The essential oils can be used in diffusers, baths, and body oils. A drop or two on a vision dream pillow, somewhere away from the eyes, may allow the answer you seek to come to you while you sleep. Dreams have always played a big part in humankind's spiritual quest. When praying, if you place the palms of your hands together, you may like to try putting one drop of your chosen essential oil on one palm, rubbing your hands together, and gently inhaling the fragrance. Some spiritual traditions do this, using powdered incense. Holding a fragrance in front of the nose helps the mind focus and concentrate. Perhaps it was this aroma-holding position that led to the tradition of holding the hands together near the face when praying.

With time and experience a person can create many different spiritual blends of essential oils for use during particular occasions, times of day, or moods. More important though, in a sense, is to have just one fragrance blend that facilitates you making the spiritual connection. This one fragrance can return you to your spiritual haven at any time, reinforcing its spiritual connotation and meaning. The aroma then becomes synonymous with the place, and to reexperience it even when out and about, at work, or when traveling, all you have to do is pull out a tissue with the blend on it, close your eyes, and sniff deeply. Instantly you can return to that spiritual place — which you experience actually within yourself. This same action, of taking your favorite fragrance with you, on a handkerchief or tissue, or in a bottle, can of course be done with a single essential oil, if you have one that is particularly effective in making the spiritual connection for you. Whether from a blend or single essential oil, the fragrance of your choice opens the door instantly to another place.

Experiment with blends, varying the proportions, as well as the essential oils. It's amazing what a drop or two, less or more, will do to a blend. If it doesn't resonate with you, discard it and start again, until you get the formula right. By "right," I mean what *you* know is right. It is not easy to blend such a special oil, so be prepared to put some time into the process. Eventually some fragrance will strike a chord in you, so just be patient and keep trying.

When blending, try to clear all thoughts out of your mind, and all ego, and instead radiate love, empathy, and compassion. I say "try" because this is not always easy to do. There is help on hand, however, and sometimes in quiet moments of love and compassion I feel the presence of angels, who help me blend together spiritual fragrances. They are out there, and they can be asked to help.

Angels have their own aromas, and they can be very difficult to replicate with earthbound fragrance. The fragrance of a particular guardian who helps me has eluded me for years. I've smelled aromas that seem similar but never exactly the same. The closest smell to it that I have found came from a bunch of magnolia blossoms given to me in a class. The aroma was rich and highly perfumed, and it gave me an immediate emotional impact. No one else present had the same reaction, because for them it did not have the same connotation. We all perceive aroma differently on a spiritual level, just as taste differs between us, and we hear sound differently, and respond to light and color in differing ways. Everything is vibration, interacting in a complex way, so choose what harmonizes with you.

The aromas we create reach out and meet those from the fragrant heavens, like the fingers of two hands mingling, making that connection we all seek. There are many types of spiritual fragrance, as individual as we are. I have my own special fragrance blend that informs my mind it is time to be still and quiet and focus on the important things — on the joy of being alive — and tells me it is time to be at peace.

MEDITATION

In a talk at the Holy Names College, in Oakland, California, Sogyal Rinpoche, a master of Dzogchen Buddhism, told a story about a man, a top diplomat and maharaja, who sought the answer to the question "How do I meditate?" He asked the question of Sogyal Rinpoche's master many times, as is the practice, to elicit many perspectives on the subject. At a spiritual dance in Sikkim, the diplomat asked the master the question again. The master was enjoying himself and replied impatiently, "Look, when one thought has ceased and died, before another thought has yet risen, isn't there a gap?" "Yes," the diplomat said. "Prolong it. Prolong that gap. That is meditation," the master explained.

A great number of books have been written on meditation, and I have written about it myself in *The Fragrant Mind*. Basically, it's very simple: Meditation is trying to create stillness and peace in the mind, beyond the usual chatter and clutter that usually fills it. This is not to say meditation is about *nothing*. To the contrary, it is about *everything*.

In meditation, we come into contact with a vast reservoir of energy, passing through ever deeper layers of ourselves, as here explained by a Tantric nun:

> The human mind is on a continuum. There's the mind, the senses — our attraction or aversion to someone or something; then there is the intellect — the everyday computer, with memory; then the creative layer — where we go deep into the mind, and there is a flow, rather than the black and white, and a deeper than bookish knowledge. The next layer is intuition, expanded awareness, where you can really distinguish between what is right or wrong and, going deep, make good decisions. The next level is the spiritual level — the sense of Oneness. The last layer is samadhi, which is complete merger in cosmic consciousness, total reabsorption. Human beings can complete the cycle: from infinite consciousness — to manifestation — to infinite consciousness.

In meditation, fragrance provides something spiritual to focus on — and with eyes closed, which many people find additionally helpful. It's important though that the aroma evokes no memory for you, which will just flood your mind and defeat the purpose of the exercise. For this reason, I suggest using blends in which no one ingredient dominates, and a new and unique aroma is created. This is accomplished by balancing out the ingredients so that even if you do not use equal drops, as some essential oils are stronger than others, there is balance between them all.

Among the floral essential oils, linden blossom, jasmine, and rose maroc make particularly good meditation oils, either individually or in blends. Some people might find these aromas too heavy, particularly as they progress with meditation, when the lighter, softer florals, such as rose otto, neroli, or diluted jasmine may feel more appropriate. Any essential oil can be lightened by diluting it.

Which essential oils are chosen is entirely a matter of personal preference. Some people are drawn to the resins, such as frankincense, myrrh, benzoin, styrax, copal, or one of the many balsams found throughout the world. A nice addition to any of these are the citrus-type eucalyptus lemon (*E. citriodora*) and litsea cubeba. These two generally work better in meditation blends than do the more usual citrus fruit oils. Blends are excellent for meditation, and there are many essential oils you can choose from to create your own. See the following chart for examples.

ESSENTIAL OIL BLENDS FOR MEDITATION
Invigorating Woods
Cypress, Fir, Pine, Spruce
Contemplative Woods
Amyris, Guaiacwood, Ho-wood, Sandalwood
Centering Fruits
Cardamom, Lemon, Tangerine, Vanilla
Awakening Fruits
Grapefruit, Lime, Mandarin, Orange

Change your meditation blend as often as you wish. Each one will be special in its own way. Using essential oils with meditation helps bring more vivid colors, clarity, and focus to the event. Aroma during meditation can bring forth cellular or genetic memory — scenes and pictures from our past, or from times and places that are unrelated to our present life.

Many people are discouraged from meditation for the simple reason they cannot find a seating position that is both comfortable and conforms to the positions usually adopted in pictures of people meditating — with legs crossed, or with the posterior resting on the heels. It sometimes seems that one has to be uncomfortable to do it properly! This is not so. You can meditate in any comfortable seated position. But try to keep your back straight, as this helps the flow through the energy centers along the spine. If no sitting position is comfortable, and this applies to many people, just lie on the floor. The most important thing in meditation is to be relaxed.

Some people tell me that when they meditate, they fall asleep. Does it really matter? In the sleeping state we often receive information or answers to questions, as well as information about the past, present, and future.

Meditation could be said to be conscious sleeping. We are, though, more sensitive to noise at this time, and the slightest sound can have the same effect as a cannon going off nearby — it's a shock! So take the phone off the hook and do whatever else is required to ensure you get a certain amount of peaceful time. In the profound quiet of meditation we can listen to our bodies. We may find the energetic source of any ache or pain, as well as the source of our spiritual selves.

There are now countless studies that prove meditation acts upon the body by, for example, slowing the pulse rate and calming physiological and neurological processes. Less easy to demonstrate than changes in clinical conditions, but well documented in people's reports of their experiences, is that meditation opens us up to receiving information. Answers to nagging questions or just plain unsolicited wisdom comes either from the higher self, the superconscious, or universal knowledge. Meditation, then, is not about taking a rest but about taking an adventure.

Chapter 4

On Perfumed Angels' Wings

For he shall give his angels charge over thee, to keep thee in all thy ways.
They shall bear thee up in their hands, lest thou dash thy foot against a stone.
— Psalms 91:11–12

WHEN YOU'RE SITTING AROUND WITH FRIENDS and have time for a long conversation, ask if they believe in angels. It's amazing what you'll hear. On one such evening, I heard an account of a meeting with an angel, a rather handsome one it seems, in a bar in Montreal, Canada, on a cold, snowy night. Anne was sitting at a table, quite near the stage, watching a band, with her back facing the main area of the bar. Suddenly, she was overcome with the sensation of love — deep, unconditional, total love, and she could feel it emanating at a specific point in the room, first from the door, then passing the length of the bar at the rear of the room, until it stopped. She said she smiled to herself because it was so absurd. She knew, without having *seen* anyone, exactly where this person's feet stood. It was like love-radar. And she was certain of her feelings. "I knew I loved whoever was in that space, and it didn't matter whether it was a man, woman, or gorilla. That's why it was so funny — in a split second, my whole outlook on life had changed."

After a while she turned around, knowing exactly where to look of course, and saw a tall handsome man standing there. She turned back, and had another laugh to herself. This was too good to be true! When the band finished, she got up and went back to her friends at the bar in the next room. Before she knew it, the man was standing behind her. She turned around and was amazed to see gold rays coming from around his head. The man had a halo! And no one else in the room seemed to notice! It was turning into a very unusual evening.

"I think he was an angel," Anne told us. "I've never felt so relaxed with anyone. It was a level of relaxation that is far and away more absolute than with a lover, or family, or friends, or even while on my own. It was another *level* of relaxation, like I'd just come extra-alive." Of course, we all wanted to know what happened to him. Apparently, they talked for hours at the bar, and he walked her back to where she was staying. The next day she would be getting on a plane to London, while he planned to be in Los Angeles. They were going in opposite directions. "The strange thing is," she continued, "I knew we had no future, and I didn't ask for, or give, an address. I knew I'd see him in heaven, and that was enough." Very appropriately, the bar was called The Rainbow, which made him the gold at the end of the rainbow!

Some people believe in angels because they have seen them, even in some cases, before their eyes beheld them. Other people believe in angels because they have heard their voice, or smelled their sweet fragrance and known they were near. When these things happen, there is no turning back; you *believe* in angels. Accounts of meetings are often quite extraordinary, which is, when you think about it, what we might expect. Experiences are also very personal and varied, and full of love, poetry, and drama.

I met an angel twenty years ago, and so have no doubt they exist. The light and peace that angels emanate is so profoundly different from anything on earth, it's impossible to confuse it with everyday reality. The light I saw was an overwhelming luminescence, shining in rays from every pore of the figure, who was beautiful in the extreme. The sense of peace that settled upon me was amazing, and it was alive in every molecule of my being — a feeling of total love and oneness with the universe.

Meetings with angels are a joyful gift, and a source of inspiration, and I know they've given people much to draw on. I have no idea why the illuminated one visited me in my home at that time. I had not asked to see one and did not particularly need comfort — at least not that I was aware of. Perhaps that first angel came just so I could know angels exist. Certainly the memory has been there for me to draw strength from, particularly when there have been obstacles to overcome, and it will be there for me in the future. As well as the deeper certainty they bring, angels also look out for our immediate physical safety. I know I've been helped many times by angelic beings, like one day when I was driving along, one whispered "pull over" in my ear, which turned out to be excellent advice.

I'm particularly grateful for one experience that happened during my vacation some years ago. A group of us were sitting together, with a high sand-dune barrier between us and the beach, which was some distance away. The red flag was up, and we'd been advised the sea was dangerous that day. With my three-year-old playing with friends, being looked out for by their parents nearby, I lay on my front, put my head on my arms, and, without realizing it, drifted off to sleep. I was awakened by a voice that said just one word: "sea." It was not a loud voice, or a particularly insistent one, but it had me on my feet in an instant and flying like the wind to the seashore. My feet didn't seem to touch the ground. I reached the water just as an enormous wave poised itself over my little girl, who just stood there watching the watery crest above her, oblivious to the danger. I grabbed her in my arms, pulled her away, and thanked the voice from the bottom of my heart.

I'm inclined to believe an angel whispered that word in my ear, rather than say it was "intuition," because I have seen a shining being standing in my own living room and *that* wasn't intuition! Angels are very physical at certain times, and very etheric at others. They straddle the two universes. My experience of them accords with the current theological position that, according to Canon Emeritus of Ely Cathedral, describes "angels as spiritual beings intermediate between God and mankind." He adds that it's thought angels were created before humankind, and because they were somehow implicated in the Creation's Fall from Perfection, there are "fallen angels." In *New Catholic Encyclopaedia*, angels are described as "celestial spirits who serve God in various capacities." Pope John Paul II has stated that angels do exist and that they "have a fundamental role to play in the unfolding of human events."

Religious literature abounds with accounts of angels, who presumably went around helping people in ancient times too. They feature strongly in the Bible and the Koran, and they're known as *devas* or "shining ones" in Hinduism. The sacred mountain of Kangchenjunga, on the border of Nepal and Sikkim, is known as "the five thrones of the Shining Ones." There are also Native American accounts of "shining beings" who advise during vision quests, and stories about "the feathered people" and "the winged ones." In European art, angels grace the corners of innumerable religious paintings, put there by Renaissance and other artists who believed implicitly in their existence. In countless towns and villages in Europe, angels carved in stone have been built into the fabric of medieval and later churches to protect the congregation within.

> *But verily over you*
> *(Are appointed angels)*
> *To protect you,*
> *Kind and Honourable,*
> *Writing down (your deeds)*
> *They know (and understand)*
> *All that ye do.*
> — Koran, Sura 82:10–12

In my experience, angels have a fragrance that precedes their "appearance," or remains after they have left. Perhaps the fragrance was also there when I actually saw the angel, but was "cut out," as my senses focused intently on the vision in front of me. I tried really hard to remember each visual detail, and was mesmerized by what appeared to be wings. Each "feather" seemed to be a center or vortex of energy made up of light, the spine in particular being a source of great light, yet also a route to the infinite, while each delicate strand coming off it was a chain made up of many sparkling lights. Each sparkle on each strand had its own energy field, and together they made the form of each superluminous "feather," which was less a material feather than an arrangement of light in a feather shape. The overall effect was extremely powerful and awe-inspiring.

I've found the fragrance of angels elusive in the sense that it seems to have no source. It's nonlocal. It just suddenly appears and suffuses the whole body and mind. I can recall two aromas quite distinctly, neither of which I have encountered before. One was fairly similar to a heavy, deep, exotic rose maroc. The other was a light fragrance that was sweet and floralish, but not just a floral, also a resin. Imagine frankincense as a flower but without the same aroma. Sometimes I will smell an angel without seeing one, and I know it is the fragrance of an angel because it's so pervading and fills my nose to the point that I feel I can't take the fragrance or inhale any longer.

After such powerful aromatic experiences, I always look carefully and sniff around to see if there was any other possible source for the phenomenon. I check my clothes for perfume and my essential oil store for any open bottles or spills. I sniff all the plants and flowers, and run through my mind who has been in the house possibly wearing scent, but no source for the strange fragrances has ever been found. Others in the house have smelled it too, and the mystery remains long after the fragrance has gone.

People who report fragrance associated with angel visitations invariably say the aroma is like jasmine, rose, lily, hyacinth, or violets. Personally, I expect people use these descriptions because the actual smell is impossible to describe — as we have nothing to compare it to on earth — and the fragrance of these particular flowers is as close as we can get. I've also smelled something *like* the aroma of freesias, but not quite. We should not expect the fragrance of the angels to reflect what is here on earth, as the angels are of heaven, not earth. Indeed, as H. C. Moolenburgh, MD, has commented in *A Handbook of Angels*, "I think at times we take in the perfume of the angel hierarchies themselves."

Fragrance is one of the sacred codes of the celestial heavens. We can in some sense consume the aroma of angels like angel food, an etheric manna from heaven, which is also angelic illumination. At the same time, fragrance invites the angels toward us, and acts as a celestial go-between. As light is contained within fragrance, it is a means by which we can communicate, a form of light transference that carries our message to the illuminated realms. Sometimes the fragrance of angels is overpowering, at other times it is barely perceptible, like a breath exuding a heavenly fragrance that only briefly touches the skin, a lightness ethereal but tangible. Perhaps to smell an angel is to be kissed by the Divine.

If angels are a link between the minds of man and God, fragrance is one language we speak. Fragrance stimulates and releases truth, opening our higher selves, making us receptive to angels as we vibrate more spiritually, aligning our energy more closely with the angelic realm. The energy of angels is very powerful, so powerful that in most instances our feeble human bodies could not withstand the force of their presence. Angels vibrate at such a high rate that their frequency could easily fragment or immobilize us. The individual guardian angels that have been assigned to us may have the means to tap into our mortal frequency, with a little help from us in the form of prayer, right thinking, love, and, perhaps, certain fragrances that put us in a state of spiritual grace. Perhaps when we are vibrating at a low emotional level, with anger, fear, hostility, and guilt, they cannot come into contact with us for reasons to do with our own safety — or predestination — and can only stand by or help from a distance, invisible to us.

Today, all over the world, people are speaking openly about their experiences with angels, who assist people with warnings or rescues, and offer consolation in difficult times. Some people are realizing that angels are our co-workers in positivity, although for others, angels remain the stuff of legends and fairy tales. Our perceptions are colored not only by culture but by experience. Angels may come as a waking vision, in a dream state, by the whiff of a celestial aroma, by a sound, or merely by a feeling of presence.

Acknowledgment is important. If we tell ourselves angels are not real, then they will not be. If we consciously dismiss angels as something from a bygone era, they may not show themselves to us. With their unconditional love, they may not wish to disturb our chosen life view. This isn't to say they're not going to help us; they do the work anyway. But if we consciously or even subconsciously exclude them, it makes it harder for them to cross over to the physical plane and help us. To give help, they need our willingness to receive it.

Once you start connecting with angels, you'll notice they're everywhere. From being "blind" to angels, you suddenly notice them on cards or in architecture — and even in real life. Angels do not have to prove their existence to us. Angels are the thoughts of God manifested. When we can all connect through the spark of love in our hearts, then the angels will be visible. When we all hold the divine spark of unconditional love, then the earth will glow and the work of the angels will be done.

We may well smell angels, or see angels looking, as we expect them to, as designed by our cultural beliefs. In the Christian tradition they usually appear as sparkling white with wings, or they come in golden splendor, with halos. This may be an aspect of what Native Americans call "shift changing" or "shape changing," the ability to change etheric shape, and change kinetic energy into dynamic energy. The same angel energy may come to different people in different forms, as our intellect will accept. It may be seen in human form and shining white light, or gold. It may have two wings, or four, or six, or none, or big enfolding wings like a dove. Some people may see colorful robes of deep blue or turquoise, or of silver and gold. Some may see an intense diffuse light and no form as such. Some smell a fragrance, many do not. Some people simply sense a presence and call it, if not "an angel," "my guardian angel," or "my guardian spirit," "spirit guide," "spiritual keeper," or a "messenger" or "traveler." These words may describe a whole world of etheric beings that exist between humans and the deity, or they may all be manifestations of the same thing. One thing is sure: There's *something* out there, and it's looking after us.

> There are also celestial bodies, and bodies terrestrial: but the glory of the
> celestial is one, and the glory of the terrestrial is another.
>
> — 1 Corinthians 15:40

Angels weave in and out of human existence, their missions to perform in countless different ways. Any dictionary of angels has so many entries, with so many names and events, it seems there have been many human-angel interactions over the years. Angels have been ascribed to nations, fire, water, earth, air, wind, hurricanes, tornadoes, earthquakes, lightning, and comets, and to strength and beauty, as well as to plants, herbs, fruits, trees, and animals.

> And, behold, there was a great earthquake: for the angel of the Lord
> descended from heaven, and came and rolled back the stone from the
> door, and sat upon it. His countenance was like lightning, and his raiment
> white as snow.
>
> — Matthew 28:2–3

The appearance of angels can be dramatic, as above, when an angel rolled back the stone from the door of the sepulcher — the burial place or cave — where the body of Jesus had been laid; or as St. Paul states below, we may be unaware of who they are.

Let brotherly love continue. Be not forgetful to entertain strangers: for
thereby some have entertained angels unawares.

— Hebrews 13:1–2

In the spiritual traditions of Judaism, Christianity, Islam, and Persia, angels have been most prevalent, particularly within the mystical traditions. Indeed, over the years angels have proliferated and caused major confusion among academics. Gustav Davidson, in the introduction to his *Dictionary of Angels, Including the Fallen Angels*, says he became overwhelmed by the sheer number of angels that appeared in the literature, which ". . . yielded a boundless profusion of angels (and demons), and I soon had more of the fluttering creatures than I knew what to do with." No doubt some of the fallen angels, or "dark angels" (those without light), as they are sometimes called, can be accounted for as people found excuses for things they had done wrong — "the fallen angel made me do it" syndrome. But there is another dimension to this subject, which the Anglican priest and author Dr. Martin Israel interpreted thus for the TV program *Network First*:

> I doubt whether anything defies the divine fiat. I think God created
> dark angels like the light angels. The dark angels are here to make us
> grow on through our own experience in life. We have to undergo
> darkness as well as light to grow as people.

The roots of many religions can be found in angel visitations. *The Book of Mormon* is based on "the gospel of a new revelation" — laws written on gold tablets that lay buried on a hill near Manchester, a village near Lake Ontario in New York State — until their whereabouts were revealed by the Angel Moroni to Joseph Smith in 1823. He described Moroni:

> Not only was his robe exceedingly white, but his whole person was
> glorious beyond description, and his countenance truly like light-
> ning. The room was exceedingly light, but not so very bright as
> immediately around his person.

Moroni can be seen atop many contemporary Church of Jesus Christ of Latter Day Saints "temples," with trumpet in hand. The New Jerusalem Church follows the teachings of the eighteenth-century Swedish mystic and theologian Emanuel Swedenborg, who wrote of angels he had seen in human form "a thousand times" : "I have conversed with them as man to man, sometimes with one alone, sometimes with many in company." Mary Baker Eddy, who founded the Christian Scientists, wrote: "They are celestial visitants, flying on spiritual, not material, pinions. Angels are pure thoughts of God, winged with truth and love, no matter what their individualism may be."

In an introduction to one edition of the Koran, N. J. Dawood writes: "For Muslims it is the infallible word of God, a transcript of a tablet preserved in heaven, revealed to the Prophet Mohammed by the Angel Gabriel." Their first encounter took place as the prophet either slept or was in a trance, while in a cave on a mountain in spiritual retreat, and the Koran was transmitted over a period of time. So important was Gabriel to Islam that the five pillars of belief include angels: "But it is righteousness — To believe in God, And the last day, And the angels, And the Book, And the messengers" (Sura 2:177).

One well-known prayer speaks of angels: "May Michael be at my right hand and Gabriel at my left, before me Uriel and Raphael, and above my head the divine presence of God." Kabbalah, the mystical tradition of Judaism, teaches that angels are God's messengers and can turn themselves into different "shapes" — forms and manifestations.

In the New Testament, Joseph, on learning that his fiancée, Mary, was pregnant, and "not willing to make her a public example, was minded to put her away privately." The story continues: "But while he thought on these things, behold, the angel of the Lord appeared unto him in a dream, saying, Joseph, thou son of David, fear not to take unto thee Mary thy wife; for that which is conceived in her is of the Holy Ghost. And she shall bring forth a son, and thou shalt call his name Jesus. . . ." In the book of Luke, the Angel Gabriel had told Mary the same thing. News of Jesus' birth was spread by the shepherds, who had been told Jesus was "a Savior" by an angel: "And the angel said unto them, Fear not: for, behold, I bring you good tidings of great joy. . . ."

Throughout the Bible, accounts of angels abound. In the Old Testament, Jacob has a dream in which he sees a ladder between earth and heaven, with "the angels of God ascending and descending on it"; and an angel even leads people into battle: "Behold, I send an Angel before thee, to keep thee in the way, and to bring thee into the place which I have prepared."

Although angels are closely associated with Judeo-Christian and Muslim traditions, they exist in other parts of the world too. In southern Australia, the "Great Spirit" of aboriginal myth goes by the name of Nepelle, and he has a "messenger," Nurunderi. In western Ireland, the late Irish poet George W. Russell described meeting beautiful "Shining Beings" and "Opalescent Beings." He believed this latter group were what the pre-Christian Irish people called "gods":

... There was at first a dazzle of light ... this came from the heart of a tall figure with a body apparently shaped out of half-transparent or opalescent air, and throughout the body ran a radiant electrical fire, to which the heart seemed the center. Around the head ... there appeared flaming wing-like auras. From the being itself light seemed to stream outward in every direction; and the effect left on me after the vision was one of extraordinary lightness, joyousness, or ecstasy.

When we meet angels the feeling is so "out of this world," it cannot be confused with any other day-to-day mind event, or dreaming experience. I asked Anne, the woman who met an angel in the bar in Montreal, "Did you imagine it?" She said, "Look, out of all the things that have ever happened to me in my life, that was the *most* real. What happened that day was very deep, and very wise, more wise than I could dream up!" This aspect of the experience, receiving knowledge, sometimes with no words being exchanged, is too extraordinary to attribute to imagination. There are only two alternatives: Either there is an angel within, that emerges and floods us with visions, profound wisdom, and infinite peace, or there are angels without. Or, maybe, there are both.

ANGELIC AROMAS: THE ANGELIC VIBRATIONS

Angels are able to utilize the vibrational effects of fragrance, perhaps because this is the closest thing the physical world can offer to their vibration. It may be the frequency they recognize and are drawn to, rather than the smell itself. By utilizing the fragrances of nature with clear intent and purpose, it is possible to use essential oils to bring angels closer to us. In today's world, we need to be able to contact the messengers so they can assist us with our spiritual growth and send our prayers and messages of love out into the universe.

We need to let ourselves and others understand that the majority of people on the planet want peace, love, and compassion, and that we are not all driven by greed, ego, and bitterness. If the angels, or shining ones, are willing to help us, shouldn't we take the thread of light offered to us, grasp it within our hearts, and give praise and thanks for such help?

Contacting angels is not as simple as using a fragrance. Think of it like this: The angel is the driver of a bus traveling to different realms. Fragrance is the route the bus travels. It puts us on the right track, but we need to signal as well. At a bus stop this is done by putting out an arm. When using fragrance the signal is a mental one, and so when using angelic vibrations, we need to use prayer, meditation, and good intent and purpose.

Angels are not the destination, but the route. They do not travel our journey for us, they only assist us on our way. They are not there to do everything for us, so don't ask, "Please will you clear away my doubts and fears," but rather, ask, "Please be close while I deal with my doubts and fears."

A particular angel has been assigned to us, and to be able to get on its wavelength, as far as is humanly possible, we need to find our angel's or guardian's vibrational fragrance. If you have already smelled it, that makes it somewhat easier, but we can *never* make a copy of that fragrance by using substances that are of this earth. Let that be understood. We can only get as close as we can to it.

If there was a flower or plant that produced an essential oil with a vibration that always attracted angels, we'd all be growing it. But the heavenly vibrations are different from those on earth, and to find them, the most likely route is through making blends, which have a vibration different from those generated by the plant world, as they grow on this planet individually. Once you have an idea or picture of your particular needs, and wish to send it to a messenger, experiment with making your own blends until you hit upon the right note.

What follows is a list of individual fragrances, essential oils that can then be blended. Your own soul fragrance is the one at which you vibrate, and the angel assigned to you will be able to lower its vibration to this and connect with you through it. When you find it, it's an indescribable feeling of completeness, as if you dissolve into the perfume. I've seen this happen, briefly, a few times while teaching. The look on the person's face is of ecstasy, of sheer joy and peacefulness, and youthfulness, as if years of hardship just seem to melt away. It's an unbelievable sight, like all transformations are.

THE ANGELIC FRAGRANCES

The following list is based on my own and other people's experiences of angels and their fragrance, and on the experiences of my class of Aroma-Genera students, who have been full of insight as their own life tales have unfolded. There are many other fragrances that have not been listed here, as I have no personal experience with them in how they relate to the angelic realms, nor am I aware of other people's firsthand experience with them. The information below is from real-life experience, as opposed to that of legend and mythology, and although one cannot say how it works, it certainly seems to work for many people.

Do not pray directly to angels. They are messengers, fellow servants of universal good. However, we can ask them for support, with the right intent. Angels join with us on both spiritual and earthly matters. Although we may feel in need of them most strongly when tragedy strikes or sorrow envelops us, angels are also there to share in our times of happiness, positivity, and joy.

THE ANGELIC FRAGRANCES AND THEIR PROPERTIES

ANGELICA SEED

Is named after angels, many of whom are associated with the plant in legend. Its aroma can be used by those who feel uncertain, or spiritually neglected, and in this respect need to call upon their personal angel. It seems to have more effect when blended with other fragrances.

BASIL

Assists in awakening, awareness, and understanding. It allows the clearance of a muddled mind that puts up a barrier to contacting angels.

BAY

Brings the angels of our future closer. It can assist us in looking forward, particularly if we tend to dwell on what has been rather than look forward to what is to come. It can create a positive note that enables assistance to be given. Allows us to see ahead and plan for that rainy day.

BENZOIN

Enables the spirit to receive blessings. It enables us to learn the joy in receiving as well as in giving, and of the interchange of spiritual energy that takes place.

BERGAMOT

Can clear away the fogginess that often muddles us, so allowing the higher spiritual self to become attuned to our helpers. This has no specifics attached, except it is a receiver.

BIRCH

Assists in struggles of a spiritual kind, clearing away the physical barriers that impede us by keeping us from seeking the truth.

BLACK CURRANT

Assists in fearful situations, perhaps helping us to recognize elements of ourselves we would rather not face. For learning to forgive and being less judgmental.

THE ANGELIC FRAGRANCES AND THEIR PROPERTIES (CONT.)

BLACK PEPPER

Is a protective fragrance that, when used with the right intent and purpose, allows our guardian angels to bring protective elements into our lives. It can also help us when we are fearful of reuniting ourselves with spiritual aspects of life after long-term neglect.

BROOM

Assists in harmonizing our mind, body, and higher self, and in our receiving insight.

CARAWAY SEED

Is another seed oil that has protective properties, and it enables our angels to assist us in viewing our life in a spiritual light rather than a physical one.

CARDAMOM

Allows the spiritual to become interwoven with the physical. In some cases, it clears the mind sufficiently for our guardian to give us insights into how we can improve our spiritual welfare.

CARNATION

Has a scent of the angelic realm; some report it as being close to their angel's fragrance. It should be used sparingly, to open us up to receive spiritual insight, clarity, and compassion.

CARROT SEED/TOP

Is used for visions, and the realms that assist in vision quests.

CEDARWOOD

Brings the angels of wisdom closer. For purification. For the angels that watch over, helping and assisting us when in need, and to permit their vibration to come closer when the wisdom of the ages is required.

CHAMOMILE ROMAN

Touches the inner child, the delicate spirit that needs to be reconnected with the divine angels of the highest order. To bring inner peace and joyfulness.

CINNAMON

Is joyful. Encourages us to explore when we step with uncertainty and need assurance that help is at hand if we need it.

THE ANGELIC FRAGRANCES AND THEIR PROPERTIES (CONT.)

CISTUS

Can be used when a person is experiencing disconnection from the spiritual self, bringing fear. It can connect to the spiritual realms with ease and bring the whole being into balance. Sometimes associated with the visitation of angels as a strong, overpowering aroma.

CLARY SAGE

Gently awakens the angelic realm of the subconscious, bringing harmony and purpose. For the times when we pray for assistance from the angels to reveal our purpose or to at least understand a little of why we tread such a path.

CLOVE

For when we are afraid and in need of angelic assistance or at least need to believe they are close by. To send with joy our thanks to these realms in celebration.

CORIANDER

Is a signal of new life. Useful when praying for guidance and assistance while we tackle a new job or try to change an area of our lives.

CYPRESS

For when we are grieving. During bereavement this fragrance brings the angels to console us, and assist in the transition and release from the earthly love that can sometimes attach too strongly to the departed.

DILL

Brings together all the current aspects of life; for the breath of life. To look at areas of painful emotion. Can be used in vision quests to bring inner understanding.

FENNEL

Assists in physical matters, keeping the mind stable and functional, yet uplifted. To remain grounded, and to help understand the lessons to be given in this lifetime.

FRANKINCENSE

Aligns with the spiritual; a "calling" perfume. To call upon the divine orders, and to send love and prayers. Also for protective elements. To assist in keeping the heart pure and full of understanding.

THE ANGELIC FRAGRANCES AND THEIR PROPERTIES (CONT.)

GERANIUM

Will allow us to be centered enough to bring the angelic realms closer for comfort and reassurance. It contains an aroma that assists in understanding both the opportunities and disappointments that may come our way.

GINGER

Is a fragrance that brings stimulation and protection. Its courageous and fearless fragrance can be used when we need to be stimulated into action but lack the courage to do it, and so brings into our aura a strengthening energy that is transmitted by our guardians.

GRAPEFRUIT

To rejoice for the upliftment of the angelic realms in joyful appreciation. Clears the pathways to direct connection with a messenger, energizing the subconscious connections.

HELICHRYSUM — ITALIAN EVERLASTING

For persistence, endurance, and courage, enabling the path ahead to be clearer. To gain awareness of the potential dangers and pitfalls of life.

HYACINTH

Is another flower of the angelic realms that is reminiscent of many descriptions of angelic odors. It can be used when we find it difficult to express ourselves and need consolation and assurance that we are not alone and help is always nearby, if it is the will of God.

HYSSOP

For the removal of emotional uncleanliness and assistance in the expansion of the protective beings, but very much on the physical plane, assisting in the removal of the heritage of guilt and fear miasms of a psychological nature. Purifying for those who believe they have sins that must be forgiven.

JASMINE

Is a favorite of the angelic realms. Often a similar, but not the same, fragrance heralds the angels' arrival and departure. A fragrance of the shining light-beings. For assistance in love, compassion, and purpose.

JUNIPER

For assistance during purification, perhaps after nightmares or such like. It can be used during meditation to help bring the beings of light into the setting, and to understand why negative experiences may be troubling us.

THE ANGELIC FRAGRANCES AND THEIR PROPERTIES (CONT.)

LAVENDER

Awakens harmony. It's a vibration that brings the angels of compassion closer when we are in need of comfort and companionship and recognition that help is always available to us and that we are never alone.

LEMON

Is vitalizing and purifying to the mind, body, and soul. It allows directness and clarity in prayer. Angels often use this vibration to send feelings of happiness and calmness to us, to remind us to use the fertility and richness of the planet correctly.

LEMONGRASS

Is cleansing for the physical that impedes the spiritual. For times when the emotions are embedded in misery and unable to escape from it, and are in need of help to overcome it.

LINDEN BLOSSOM

For when sadness blocks the heart from feeling love, and for when we are in need of inner peace and happiness. An angelic aroma associated with angels, which brings the peace and contentment that can come only from the angelic realms.

MANDARIN

For the inner child. To reconnect with the angelic keepers of our childhood, bringing back briefly the innocence of childhood prayers.

MARJORAM

Can be used to help assist us when we become obsessive, or when we can find no relief from persistent mental anguish. It may bring assistance on an angelic level to release those holds over us.

MELISSA

Is for past life lessons and assistance in moving forward and gaining wisdom from lessons learned. For letting the angels that have accompanied you through lifetimes give you understanding and support.

MIMOSA

Comes within the angelic realms of dream states. For the angels who watch over us during the night when our soul is for a short time free of the mortal body.

THE ANGELIC FRAGRANCES AND THEIR PROPERTIES (CONT.)

MYRRH

Brings understanding and compassion, assisting wounded healers who are unable to forgive themselves. For expanding the spiritual, and to help those who are in need of energetic rescue.

MYRTLE

For forgiveness. When we wish to be forgiven and cleared of guilt and need help; when no other avenue is left open to us.

NARCISSUS

Is said to help at times of transition and to enable the angelic realms to come closer, bringing the fragrance of passing to the heavens. Often experienced by those who see angels.

NEROLI

Has the sweetness of angel's breath, the gentleness of peacefulness. It reaches the higher self and the spiritual part of our being.

NUTMEG

Brings the dreams of angelic realms into conscious thought. For assistance in physical neglect, and to slowly help in clearing away debris we no longer need.

OAKMOSS

Helps us connect with the earth plane and realize that we are on earth for a reason.

ORANGE

Brings the joy of our assigned angels into our hearts, touching us with happiness that remains within us always, if we can only acknowledge it.

PALMAROSA

Assists when we are feeling neglected or misunderstood and would like the comfort of the angelic realms.

PATCHOULI

Assists in our connection with the planet and the past vibrational patterns that we may encounter upon our journey.

THE ANGELIC FRAGRANCES AND THEIR PROPERTIES (CONT.)

PEPPERMINT

Is strong and clearing, and can be used when barriers have been erected and all help has been refused. Used to clear a pathway.

PETITGRAIN

Gives gentle awakening. This esssential oil allows us to gently awaken our consciousness and connect, if only briefly, with the subconscious and higher self, attuning with spiritual growth.

PINE

Allows the angels of nature to enter the atmosphere. For assistance during vision quests, dream states, balancing, and for holders of the star energy. Their fragrance lives on after they have left, with only their ethereal shapes and auras left behind. This connecting ability remains in the fragrance — an angel to assist in creativity that stems from the heart.

ROSE

Is a fragrance of angels that comes in various scents — some are headier, some are lighter. Rose can be used to bring our consciousness closer to our angels and to the angelic self that dwells within us. To inhale rose is to inhale the love and kisses of angels.

ROSEMARY

Brings protection when unwell. It's used to bring the healing elements of angelic beings forward, although all elements of these beings can be healing if God wishes it. It helps us recognize that we have a conscious mind, a subconscious mind, and a superconscious mind, and that we are always spiritual beings.

SAGE

For when it's difficult to understand humanity's actions and to bring the spiritual energy of the light-beings close. To purify environments, to truly connect into the spirit of our home (every home does have a heart). To bring the wisdom of the ages into our hearts.

SANDALWOOD

Assists in the joining of the physical and spiritual realms, the reaching beyond ourselves into the universal whole. For those who cannot visualize the connection between the conception of the universe and the conception of humankind.

THE ANGELIC FRAGRANCES AND THEIR PROPERTIES (CONT.)

SPIKENARD

Contacts the angels of potentiality. It expands or contracts, revealing the secrets of the soul and the light of the universe.

THYME

Is strengthening and gives courage when courage and strength are needed to overcome fear and disillusionment. For when we need to call upon the deity for physical assistance. During visions and dream states, messengers bring insights into our physical obstacles and insights of how to overcome them.

TUBEROSE

Is a fragrance associated with a particular type of angelic being — seemingly one who brings messages very clearly and with much love. The fragrance assists us in understanding our life's purpose, and perhaps in how better to give the love that we have been given in abundance from the angelic realms and God.

VERBENA

Assists us in attuning to the higher spiritual self and in attempting to complete the harmonization between mind and spirit.

YARROW

Is a fragrance for when we are in search of spiritual understanding, stimulation, and clarity. Some report that yarrow can bring answers into the mind following prayer.

YLANG YLANG

Is calming and soothing for those with troubled minds and who find it difficult to like themselves very much, or forgive themselves — but who need to forgive and to find a place in their hearts to love themselves. Aids us in looking at this wonderful world we have been given, with love and the understanding that we are all beautiful and a part of it.

Chapter 5

A Fragrant Transition

And there came also Nicodemus, which at the first came to Jesus by night, and bought a mixture of myrrh and aloes, about a hundred pound weight.
Then took they the body of Jesus, and wound it in linen clothes with the spices, as the manner of the Jews is to bury.

— John 19:39–40

ONE OF THE MOST INTERESTING QUESTIONS in life is "What happens after death?" This question is relevant not only to us, the living, but to people we have loved and who are no longer with us. We live in hope that they or their spirits live on. Each spiritual tradition has its answer to "the big question," and it's very confusing that various religions differ so much in their beliefs. Our ancestors didn't have this problem, as they usually grew up and lived within one spiritual tradition and adhered to that. Today people travel the world, watch TV programs about other cultures and beliefs, and read innumerable books — with different answers — on the subject. No wonder so many are in spiritual "crisis," unsure of where to turn, and even more uncertain about what the inevitable future will bring.

One source of information comes from "near-death experiences." People who have reported this experience are remarkably similar in their reports. First, they say, the spirit floats above the dead body, watching doctors or other people trying to revive it, and hearing all that goes on. Then they see a bright white light, or a tunnel appearing before them. At the end of this tunnel, or on the other side of a river, there is someone to greet them, variously described as a lone figure shining brilliantly, an angel, Jesus, a spiritual guide, or beloved family members and friends, even pets. Whatever the differences in these accounts, one thing is constant — the profound sense of peace that envelops these people; they often don't want to return to this life, but are told their time has not yet come. These near-death experiences are often associated with fabulous fragrances, which are described as "heavenly," "delicious," "unbelievable," and "indescribable."

Fragrance plays a unique part in the interfaces, not only between the living and their earlier lives but between the living and the dead, and between the present and past lives. Indeed, aroma is a language that traverses many layers of existence, an avenue not only of exploration but of explanation.

The most common of these aromatic revelations occurs between people who have died and people they loved who have been left behind. The following story was told to me by a client: "I used to live with this man and loved him very much, but he left me, and I never heard from him again. That had been a long time ago. Then one evening I drove past a road that led to where he lived, and I had a very strong urge to drive past his house. I fought the feeling, but it was so difficult that I felt torn apart. I hadn't thought about him for ages but now, all of a sudden, he flooded my mind. I was at traffic lights, telling myself to be strong and not to even think about driving past the house. The lights changed and I drove home. All the way, I had a deep emotional sensation, remembering how good we had been together, and I felt the hurt all over again. Suddenly, the emotion changed, and I felt flooded with love.

"The next day I had almost forgotten about the incident and was getting on with my work, when I smelled his aftershave. It was an unusual one he'd had sent over from Italy. It was in my nose, and everywhere I went I could smell it. Suddenly, I knew he'd died and passed on, and this was his way of saying good-bye and that he had really loved me. I cried for a while but the smell kept hitting me, again and again, and the love filled me. I must have fallen asleep in the chair, and when I woke up there was no smell. All the pain and hurt I'd felt for years had gone. I knew then I could find someone else because before that I'd always been alone, afraid of being hurt again. His passing and sending me love made me realize I'm lovable, that I deserve to find another person, and that my life could start again."

Stories of aromas particularly associated with a person who has passed on are not uncommon. It is sometimes the smell of flowers that the loved one liked or that the deceased used to give to the person left behind. There are other smells we might associate with a person, such as perfume or tobacco smoke, and workplace odors — coal in relation to a coal miner, for example — and the smell of food, such as garlic, a person particularly liked. The more general aromas of people are also found lingering in the air, and these aromas may be quite imperceptible to other people. But, more commonly, the aroma is simply a powerful floral fragrance with no particular connotation to either the recipient or the person who has transcended the earthly experience.

Fragrances that occur at times of bereavement bring with them memories and comfort. Perhaps they are brought by angels, so we know that person is at one with the heavens and is sending this message of love. Perhaps the spirit has come to say good-bye, to let us know it is there in the ether and is moving on. Some would say it is just the mind playing tricks, but it is not just the aroma that comes. Associated with it is information that is often as clear as a bell, and comes not from within, but from without. The fragrance is reassuring because it is a link, but it is also transformational in that it can jolt us out of a behavioral mold, allowing us to move on, and in some sense we are released.

This experience of "scenting" happened to a Mrs. Case of Exeter, England, who then went on to research the subject. In *Odour of Sanctity*, the private publication that resulted, she wrote:

> People who have lost their sense of smell can smell it. Sometimes
> two people can smell it, and a third cannot. Sometimes many people
> share it; and often, as in a service in church, only one person smells
> it and the others notice nothing. Sometimes the scent is diffused, and
> at others localized.

One of her informants, a widow, wrote: "I felt dreadful all that day and eventually prayed for the phenomena of scentings and warmth to return and next day it was back again and remained with me another week or two, gradually lessening as my burden of grief became more bearable." Mrs. Case notes that "the sanctity derives from the agent, not the recipient," meaning that these kinds of extrasensory olfactory experiences relate to ordinary human beings who have passed on to the place that produces "the odor of sanctity." This phenomenon is different from that whereby people living here on earth produce an "odor of sanctity" signifying their special holiness.

Christian saints often emitted sweet-smelling fragrances while both dead and alive. The sweet aroma of St. Patrick apparently filled the room in which his body lay. The English St. Milburga, a daughter of Merewald, prince of Mercia, founded a monastery for virgins in Wenlock and died in 700 CE. Her body lay in a vault in St. Milburga's church for four hundred years and was almost forgotten, until a sweet-smelling perfume emitting from her tomb led to its rediscovery. The seventeenth-century St. Teresa of Avila spent twenty years as a contemplative sister of the Carmelite order, then became a reformer, before dying at the age of sixty-eight. Some years later, a sweet fragrance began to come from her grave, and the body was exhumed and found to be fresh and whole.

In the twelfth century, St. Isiodore's body was disinterred forty years after his death and again four hundred years later, and both times it was found not to have decayed and to be emitting a fabulous odor. And in the early seventeenth century, the coffin of the Russian St. Juliana, when opened so one of her sons could be buried with her, was found to have a beautiful fragrance coming from it.

The Greek Orthodox St. Demetrius left relics that exuded a sweet-smelling oily substance. This phenomenon, which also occurs with icons, is known as "myrrh gushing," and the substance was said to have healing properties. A basilica was built on the site of St. Demetrius's death, and pilgrims used to collect the fragrant oil from a basin in the crypt, which can be seen to this day in Thessaloníki. The relics themselves stopped producing the oil when they were stolen by Italian crusaders in the thirteenth century, and although they were returned to Greece in 1980, the relics have not exuded it since. However, a strong fragrance is often smelled around them. A myrrh-exuding icon can be seen today at the monastery of Malevi near Tripoli, in the Peloponnese.

A great number of saints were said to be fragrant during their lives. St. Francis of Assisi is said to have smelled of lemon, St. Rose of rose, St. Catherine of violet, and St. Cajetan of orange blossom. St. Lydwyne's aroma had several components, including cinnamon, ginger, clove, rose, and violet; while the breath of thirteenth-century Blessed Herman of Steinfeld was like a garden of fragrant flowers.

This "odor of sanctity," as it is called, denotes the person has been elevated to some higher level of existence, one closer to the Divine. It puts people in a category other than that of the base, material life. The aromas have an unreal and powerful effect, seeming to break the aromatic rules — like having no apparent source. The historical records show people were concerned to point this out and explain these aromatic happenings occurred despite there being no incense, spices, fragrant ointments, or balms around. Fragrance is supposed to be of the air, but in the case of seventeenth-century Venerable Benedicta of Notre-Dame-du-Laus, she was said to be so divinely fragrant, everything she touched became perfumed. Aroma is supposed to travel downwind, but as an Indian saying goes, "The fragrance of a flower travels with the wind, but the odor of sanctity travels against the wind."

Experiences of smell phenomena are happening today, all around the world. If they only involved one person, the unusual aromas could be dismissed as the figment of an overactive imagination. But often hundreds of people are "witness" to the same aromatic event, and we can suppose that something less explicable is going on.

THE FRAGRANCE OF THE SPIRIT

> *Your spiritual fragrance transforms the atmosphere of the world like an
> incense stick transforms the atmosphere in a room. The incense stick
> spreads its fragrance regardless of the conditions and people in the room.*
>
> — Brahma Kumaris

We each have a unique spiritual fragrance that carries the vibrational frequencies of our own spirit and is in harmonic resonance with our inner self. This fragrance is completely different from that produced by angels or any other heavenly beings. These personal spirit fragrances seem to comprise various smells, such as deep, rich resins, fully flavored fruits, fully open flowers, and verdant grasses, meadows, trees, or woods, although they are unlike any fragrances on earth and, like angel fragrances, are difficult to describe. Each fragrance has a complexity of highs and lows that weave in and out of each other, reflecting the journey of our soul. It reflects all the places we have been, all the people we have been in contact with, all the emotions we have experienced, and all the personalities we have passed through — including those from other realms and, perhaps, other lifetimes. And it is the combination of all these things that comprises our spiritual perfume. We carry the smells associated with past times, just as we carry those of this lifetime, and they are all woven inextricably together, as pieces of the same aromatic cloth. Our personal spirit fragrance is the one we are most at ease with but, at the same time, it has the capacity to affect us emotionally on the very deepest levels, stirring and moving us in ways that can be exciting, provocative, illuminating, and liberating. Ultimately, our spiritual fragrance will connect with the glorious soul fragrance, an aspect of the universal whole.

MAKING THE TRANSITION

> *Though my soul may set in darkness,
> it will rise in perfect light,
> I have loved the stars too fondly
> to be fearful of the night.*
>
> — unknown

We make plans throughout our lives, and even plan our funerals, but seldom do we plan our own deaths. This is not the case with Tibetan lamas, who place great store on the abandonment of grasping, yearning, and attachment. They give everything away before death, if possible of course, so there will be no argument over the distribution of the physical possessions, which could negatively influence the next incarnation. Some, at what they consider the right time, simply close their eyes and release their spirit. In other cultures, especially nomadic ones, old people choose to be left behind if they have difficulty keeping up with the rest of the migrating tribe, and starve to death. However, most of us do not embrace or accept death in this way; we fight it tooth and nail and think that by planning for it we're giving in.

The more usual scenario is that we experience someone else dying and find ourselves making plans for the funeral, if not the death itself. Flowers are an essential part of most funeral practices, perhaps because their fragrance brings a special atmosphere to the event. When Mother Teresa died in 1997, flowers that looked like tuberose surrounded the coffin, and I wondered if this was her favorite flower and whether they had been in the room as she made the transition. Certainly, this very aromatic flower would have filled the room with its heady perfume, as essential oil of tuberose would equally have done.

Aromas are so personal, it's impossible to suggest essential oils to use at this most important time. This is the time to use fragrances we have loved, that induce in us peace and joy. If we are too weak to organize it ourselves, friends and family can be asked to get the essential oils and diffuser so that the enveloping etheric clouds of fragrance can accompany us on the journey "home."

Make sure you use pure, natural essential oils, rather than the man-made synthetics that, to the untrained eye and inexperienced nose, can be disguised to look like the real thing. If ever there was a time we returned to nature, it is this, our true nature. We all have an image perhaps of what the afterlife will be like, but one thing is almost certain, there are no man-made chemicals in heaven.

People who have died and been resuscitated, and had near-death experiences, notice delightful aromas. We will most surely breathe in the fragrant heavens as we pass over. But when we are lying there, waiting for this to happen, what do we smell? Let us hope it is not the urine of a patient in the next hospital bed, or a nurse with body odor. Even in the comfort of our own home, we may not appreciate the smell of frying coming from the kitchen. Unpleasant odors will make it harder to find any beauty there may be in death. This is the one time in life to embrace the beautiful, by thinking of the wonderful things we have done in our life, and of the special people we have known, hopefully in the company of people who shower us with their unconditional love. Sweet-smelling aromas, well chosen and sensitively used, contribute the beauty of nature to the dying experience. And in a hospital ward, it attracts people to the area, making it less lonely.

Sogyal Rinpoche, author of *The Tibetan Book of Living and Dying*, writes:

> What counts at the moment of death is whatever we have done in our lives. Help the dying person not to face death empty handed, help him or her to find meaning in his or her life, even if he or she has many regrets now he can make the end of his life meaningful. Our state of mind at the moment, a change of heart at the time of death, can influence our future and powerfully transform our karma. Our last thoughts and emotions before death have a powerful and determining effect on our immediate future. The quality of the atmosphere when we die is important. When someone is dying we should do all we can to inspire positive emotions, sacred feelings like love and compassion. . . .

If love and emotions can be expressed, and tears allowed to fall before the actual moment of death, the spirit can be released undistracted. This brings us to a very important point: if you're preparing essential oils for someone who is dying, don't think of it as a potion to draw the person back to life. No earthly fragrance can bring them back. Think of it as simply providing a pleasant atmosphere in which the person can experience transition, or as a cloud of delicious fragrance to waft over them on their inevitable way, our last parting gift.

USING ESSENTIAL OILS TO MAKE THE TRANSITION

Which essential oils you use is entirely a matter of personal choice. The essential oils are profiled in chapter 11, and you may find that or other sections of the book useful. If you like flowers, pick from the flower essences, and if they are not right for you, there are also herbs, fruits, seeds, woods, and resins to choose from. When you are happy with a fragrance or blend, you may find your perception of the aroma changes, as you are on the steps of your own soul-fragrance evolution.

Blends have a delight all of their own, and a richness that is perhaps appropriate at this time, although many people may prefer to have a single favorite fragrance that can be found in essential oil form. Here is just one suggestion:

Rose Maroc	2 drops
Jasmine	2 drops
Hyacinth	1 drop

This is quite a heavy fragrance, but if only a small amount is used, the aroma is sweeter and lighter: the strength depends on the dilutions you use. The effect will be very different if you use two or, say, eight drops in a diffuser. It is always better to use smaller amounts to begin with, then see if the person making the transition would like more.

Spritzers

One way fragrances can be used is in a "spritzer," with water and essential oils mixed together. Boil some water with the essential oils added, keeping the lid shut very tightly. The ideal tool for this is stainless steel pots used for making herbal infusions or for cooking. Allow the mixture to cool, without opening the lid, and place it in a refrigerator for twenty-four hours. When you take it out, there may still be some oil floating on top, which can be spooned off and used in a diffuser. The water that remains will have a delicate, light fragrance, ideal for spraying around the room or on the body. For those who like to use frankincense in a blend, use only a small amount, as it can overpower the rest of the fragrances when used in this way.

Hydrolats

Another way of using natural, water-based fragrance is to blend hydrolats, which are the floral waters left after distillation. Rose and orange flower (neroli) are just two of the fragrances that could be used, and are ideal for spraying rooms, bed linens, and around people, as they have antiseptic properties, as well as a delicious fragrance. However, because only the water-soluble components of the plant remain in the water, the hydrolat will not smell exactly the same as the flower. Lavender hydrolat smells not at all like the lavender we know so well, and rosemary hydrolat can be quite camphoraceous.

Fragrance and Transition — The Long Tradition

In the ancient world, fragrance was an essential element in funerary rites. In Genesis 49:33, Jacob "yielded up the ghost," and in Genesis 50:2, "Joseph commanded his servants the physicians to embalm his father." In Chronicles 16:14,

King Asa "slept with his fathers" and was laid "in the bed which was filled with sweet odors and divers kinds of spices prepared by the perfumer's art." Some versions of the Bible say "apothecaries' art." An account of the death of the Persian King Yezdijird, in 652 CE, reports he was embalmed with spices and perfumes; while the ancient Egyptians, as we know, used a great deal of fragrant material in mummification.

Fragrance had deep symbolic meaning to our ancestors, who considered it a gift of the gods. It was, indeed, seen as both an expression of the Divine and as something that conferred divinity or immortality. The fragrant sap of trees — the resins of many ancient incenses — was seen as the sweat or tears of the gods, while the unaccountable loveliness of scents from flowers and herbs were seen as tools of divine inspiration. The ancient Taoists, with their eyes ever on transformation, noted that a solid incense stick becomes, with fire, a fragrance that disappears in the air, while the ancient Roman writer Lucretius was struck by the idea that the soul is part of the body, as fragrance is part of a piece of frankincense resin. He wrote of death, "The breath of life is driven without . . . scattering abroad like smoke."

So important to the ancient Greeks was the custom of anointing the limbs of the departed with perfumed oil, they felt obliged to do this also to their greatest enemies, if there was nobody else around to do it. After a cremation, at which incense would be thrown on the fire, the bones and ashes were washed with wine, mixed with precious ointments, and placed in a funeral urn. At one point in Homer's *Odyssey*, the practice is described: "But when the flames your body had consumed, with oils and odors we your bones perfumed. . . ." According to the nineteenth-century perfumer Eugene Rimmel, "Perfumes were thought such an essential part of funeral ceremonies that scent bottles were painted on the coffins of the poorer class of people as a sort of empty consolation for the absence of the genuine article." Fragrances were daubed on the tombs, and scented flowers strewn around.

All this was too much for the writer Anacreon, who thought the precious fragrances should be enjoyed in life:

> *Why do we shed the rose's bloom*
> *Upon the cold insensate tomb?*
> *Can flowery breeze or odour's breath*
> *Affect the slumbering chill of death?*
> *No, no; I ask no balm to steep*
> *With fragrant tears my bed of sleep;*
> *But now while every pulse is glowing,*

Now let me breathe the balm flowing;
Now let the rose, with blush of fire,
Upon my brow its scent expire.
                                        — Ode 32

The most extravagant user of aromatics in ancient Rome — in death as in life — was the Emperor Nero. At his wife Poppaea's funeral, it's said that more incense was consumed than could be produced in "Arabia" in a year. As did the Greeks, the Romans put ashes and bones in urns with perfumes, and the more perfume was used, the more wealthy the departed were or the more loved they were said to be.

For thousands of years in India, the funeral pile has contained scented woods such as sandalwood, and spices and fragrant gums and resins. The main source for these materials is the town of Ghazipur, which is just upriver on the Ganges from Benares, the area's biggest market for fragrance materials and the Hindu spiritual center of India.

Muslims in Pakistan associate fragrance very closely with heaven and say that five hundred angels gather near a person who has died. Just before the body is sprinkled with scent by the attendants, the angels sprinkle perfume brought from heaven. When the soul leaves the body, it is smeared with the fragrance of Paradise and transported to heaven.

In Japan, the youngest child sets fire to a pile of fragrant woods, and fragrant materials are also thrown upon it. In China, at least until a hundred years ago, the body was perfumed, much incense was burned, and those in the funeral procession carried burning fragrant material.

The reasons for using fragrance when making the transition are many, including the idea that the rising of the smoke literally carries the spirit of a person to higher realms. Because sweet-smelling fragrance was so strongly associated with the heavenly realms, a person was expected to be aromatically acceptable when he or she arrived there. It was through aroma the dead and eternal met.

Muslims of the Indian subcontinent have traditionally burned incense, which might include benzoin, sandalwood, or patchouli, in an *oodsoz*, or "censer," and this is lit at the moment of death and placed by the feet of the body. In the United Arab Emirates, perfuming the body is done partly so the deceased should be sweet-smelling when meeting God, but also because fragrance is said to attract angels and banish evil spirits. This idea has been, and continues to be, very widespread, right across the world.

Not everyone can bear the idea of dying, and you can understand why. The Chinese in particular have a long tradition of seeking "the herb of immortality" or "the fungus of immortality," and many great tales have been written around characters who made the heroic attempt to locate them. Describing one such "Gold Medicine," in 400 CE, is Ko Hung (Pao Pu Tse):

> The medicine should be prepared on a famous mountain...The compounder...should perfect the purification and ointment of the body with the five perfumes...when the medicine is made, not only will the successful manipulator be immortal, but all the rest of his family will become immortal as well.

Chapter 6

Remembrance of Fragrance Past

The details of burial, the herb that was used to ward off sickness, and the statues of gods are all typical of classical regression.
— Dr. Brian Weiss, *Through Time into Healing*

MEMORIES ARE IN OUR CELLS, or in the spaces between them, or in their electromagnetic field, or their aura. Cellular memory has long been reported by bodyworkers such as aromatherapists, reflexologists, and rolfers, as well as shiatsu, kinesiology, acupressure, and connective tissue massage (CTM) therapists, among others. During bodywork, when certain parts of the body are being manipulated, earlier events in this life, and in some cases "past" lives, are often released and recalled.

A different perspective has been put on this subject by heart and lung transplant patient Claire Sylvia, author of *A Change of Heart*. At the age of forty-eight, after the transplant, she developed a new liking for chicken and beer, and experienced the sensation that another person was within her. In a dream, she met "Tim L.," who after some research she discovered was in fact the young man whose organs had been donated to her following a fatal motorcycle accident.

These two dimensions to the subject of memory are interesting enough, but there are more. Richard is a lighting engineer for an American ballet company and was on tour with the troupe in Germany. The bus stopped for a break at a rest stop near a village, and Richard came out to stretch his legs. He felt drawn to walk down a path between two houses, until he came to a pond. At this point he can't remember what happened, but the others told him later. Apparently, he'd started shouting and yelling and waving his arms about, obviously very distressed. Some residents came out of their houses and figured he must have something to do with the coach, and they brought his companions to the scene. Richard was speaking German, a language he had never studied, and explained to the coach driver, who was German and spoke the language, that he was a

German soldier drowning in the pond, having fallen through the ice. There are tens of thousands of recorded cases of people experiencing other lives, many of them including *xenoglossy*, the ability to speak fluently in a foreign language without having learned it in this lifetime.

These feelings, of having died in another place and time, happen to children too. I can think of one little girl living in rural Ireland who remembered being hit by a truck on a road in America, a place she'd never been, and described the red and white logo on the side of the truck perfectly. The parents were intrigued by this as they lived a very simple life without TV or Coca-Cola, and the girl was not familiar with American culture, yet alone place-names. They subsequently took their daughter to the United States to confirm the details. Another little girl, who was three at the time, told me she'd left a family behind and didn't "belong" in her current family. Suddenly, like a window into another world, she stopped being three and, speaking with the vocabulary of an adult, told me she'd been a man, married with children, and had died falling off an amusement park carousel. She also gave the name of the man's wife. Then she noticed a flower, and enraptured by it, ran off and was three years old again.

Many books have been written about past-life experiences, usually those that emerge during hypnosis. There are, then, several primary methods of recall: through hypnosis; through "always knowing," as in the case of children; through suddenly realizing, as in the case of Richard; and through bodywork. But there is another route into the past, through aroma, which can bring back memories not only of earlier events in this life, but of lives experienced before.

Many contemporary religions believe in past lives, while others have in the past adhered to this doctrine but no longer do. Hinduism and Buddhism teach reincarnation, and thus past lives, saying that the soul must pass through many lifetimes, each one teaching valuable lessons, until the spirit reaches perfection and may ascend to a higher place. Rebirth was a concept long accepted in the Jewish tradition until the nineteenth century. Today it remains part of the teachings of the Hasidic sect and has continued through the mystical Judaic tradition of Kabbalah. Among Christians, it was accepted until Emperor Constantine, in 325 CE, decided to edit references to it out of the texts.

Where are the past-life memories coming from? Some would say they are not about spirit transference, that is reincarnation of one spirit into the body of a person at a later time. Rather, they say, our DNA, or the etheric energy that enfolds it, carries memories of activities/emotions experienced by our direct ancestors. Depending on whether a gene is active or recessive, we inherit hair and eye color, body shape, and other physical characteristics. But we also carry things for which no genes have been found, such as generosity, meanness, the love or fear of certain things, temperament, emotional aspects, and general approach to life. If such intangible things can somehow be replicated, perhaps there are other, energetic "genes" that carry memories and the emotions that are associated with them.

But how do we explain the visitation of "Tim L." to Claire Sylvia in the dream? Can the cell, including its associated energy field, hold the memory and behavior not only of the person up to and until the moment of death, but also the individualized "spirit" of the person?

Many questions are raised by these issues. Organ transplants give a modern twist to "other-life" existences, but basically this is an ancient subject that has played an important part in the spiritual development of people around the world, many of whom have their own bodywork systems, ways to go into a hypnotic state, spontaneous experiences, and aromatic ceremonies.

Aroma and memory are, of course, inextricably linked. The pathway for this in physical terms is from the nose, to the olfactory nerves, to the limbic system and other portions of the brain. Olfactory nerves are actually part of the brain, extending from it into the nasal cavity, where they meet aroma molecules via receptors. Nothing gets closer to the brain than aroma. The brain, we now know thanks to research in psychoneuroimmunoendocrinology, is an ongoing system, producing neurochemicals that have receptors on cells in all parts of the body, a continuum with undefined borders. Aroma induces the release of brain chemicals, and thus can "reach" or affect the whole body.

In addition, from pictures of the auric field of aromas — in the form of essential oils — we can see they have a colorful dynamism that interacts with the auric field of a person. Aromas, then, are unique in being the one physical/etherical element that appears to reach all parts of our body and, perhaps, all parts of our spirit.

Is it any wonder that smell has such a profound effect on us, or that extended memory can be triggered by certain aromas? Aroma is one of the means by which memory is laid down by its as yet mysterious recording mechanism. Aromas that have no particular association for us in this lifetime can act as a trigger, releasing the memory association that may have been laid down in a former life. The mechanism for this may be essentially physical, with the aroma molecules acting on the cells indirectly by stimulating neurosecretory hormones to act upon the cell receptors, as keys in the locks. Looking at it from an energetic viewpoint, there may be a parallel universe in which aroma is itself the key that unlocks the memory receptors. And as the etheric energy is eternal, rather than physically mortal like the flesh, the memories can relate not only to this lifetime but to other times held in the etheric field.

THE AROMA-GENERA EXPERIENCE

Aroma-Genera is a system I have developed for the release of emotions that are attached to experiences of past events, both in this lifetime and beyond. During this process, a fragrance associated with a particular personality sometimes brings to the front of the mind an experience that belongs to another time. Nine particular blends are used, and by inhaling them with eyes closed, other times are reached.

Some of the present-life memories that are recalled can seem very trivial, and they show how sensitive human beings really are. A child can be deeply hurt by a casual offhand comment, or made to feel inadequate by being unable to tie a shoelace. Even newborn babies can become traumatized, as evidenced by the case of a woman who remembered, as a newborn baby, being separated from her mother in the delivery room and put behind a curtained screen. It's frightening to think how many babies have had to undergo similar distress because adults don't understand the emotions even newborns can experience. So many hurts are being carried forward in time, unbeknown to us. Memories arise from adulthood too and reveal emotions we may have hidden even from ourselves, such as loss and fear.

Past-life memories can, unlike present-life recall, involve death. This is sometimes traumatic and sometimes not obviously so, although there is always an emotion attached. For example, one woman recalled being hung for stealing an apple. She asked, bewildered, "An apple? An apple? They'd hang me for an apple?" and it was the emotion of unfairness that clung tenaciously to her present. In another case, a man recalled a lifetime in which he was so fat that when he died his family had difficulty getting him out of his bed and down the stairs. He was very embarrassed that his dead body had continued to release horrible, smelly odors. Not coincidentally, in this lifetime he had an obsession with cleanliness or, rather, had an obsession before it was dissipated by the Aroma-Genera session.

As we know, there are often several traumatic moments in a person's life. One Native American woman with a fear of enclosed underground spaces had her fear explained during Aroma-Genera. She was a young girl of three or four waiting for a tornado to pass, with her family in the root cellar of their house.

Suddenly she got the sensation they were not safe where they were, and she told her family, who disagreed. But she was so insistent everyone eventually left the cellar, only seconds before the whole building collapsed into it. It was the meeting of the past aroma, of the cellar and roots, and the present aroma, one of the nine Aroma-Genera blends, that brought this memory out of the lifetime's memory vault. The girl and her family did not die and were not harmed by the experience, but she was still holding the fear until it was released by Aroma-Genera.

I've heard hundreds of similar stories during Aroma-Genera sessions, and am led to believe that it is the *emotions* around a particular situation that get trapped within the invisible energy field of a person — be that the electromagnetic field, the etheric field, bioplasmic field, orgone, or whatever. It is not so much the dying, or the people or circumstances of a particular memory, its magnitude or triviality, but the emotion — the core feeling behind the event or memory — that carries forward and interferes with the flow of life.

What is so clear from past-life or earlier present-life recall is that events in the past can rest in the energy, causing it to flow in the wrong direction. The past emotion sits like a rock in the river of life, sending us off course. These rocks of distortion send us into directions that relate to the past, not to the future we should enjoy unencumbered by the past. We become, as the saying goes, "bent out of shape." We are hindered by emotions such as anger, anxiety, and shame that bear no relation to the life we are living right now.

The Aroma-Genera experience is very gentle, and very releasing. No hypnotic techniques are involved. At all times the person is fully aware of the present, and also of the sensation he or she is involved in, enabling the person to discuss each step of the experience as a detached observer. Indeed, the aroma seems to allow us to straddle two time-place existences. Take for example the case of Martin, who recalled being an innkeeper at a place some distance away from London during the great fire of 1666. He described standing with his wife, watching the dramatic scene on the horizon as London burned, sending the aroma of burning wood far and wide. At one point his voice lowered and he appeared to be talking to someone. He was giving highly detailed instructions to his wife to prepare more beds and food, as they would surely be busy that night. He was having two conversations, in two times, as we might have two conversations with two people in our one time. The present-day Martin, objectively viewing his old self, was amused that he had been more interested in the monetary fortune to be gained from London burning than in the fate of the people directly involved in the fire. Interestingly, in this lifetime, Martin works as a healer with people suffering post-traumatic stress. He hypothesized that he was now making up for his past selfish behavior, and perhaps assuaging the subsequent guilt he may have felt.

Aroma-Genera is not a regression therapy. It involves working with personality types, which may be imposed on us, or adopted by us, to get us through the present-day life. However, through Aroma-Genera, personalities from somewhere else do emerge. There is always a key moment, a pivotal point that keeps coming up until its message is understood and resolved.

This is not a process that can be undergone alone, and the essential oil blends cannot be mixed together in an arbitrary way. Using aroma in such a way is a precise science. There is absolutely no need for standard regression techniques, where a person is led back in time; the aroma does that instead. Nor is there any need for hypnotism. The state induced by aroma is *not* like being regressed, or hypnotized, and neither is it like dreaming or daydreaming. Aroma takes us down another route entirely.

Aroma-Genera is a system that uses aroma like a searchlight, seeking within to find that which waits to be found. But there is another approach, that is when a particular aroma haunts a person, either in a positive way, or a negative one. For example, a person might find a particular aroma abhorrent for no apparent reason and this may be indicative of a hidden story that could be released by that aroma. In these cases, a sample of the aroma could be taken to a psychotherapist, counselor, or Aroma-Genera practitioner, or someone else professionally trained to understand the psychological process that goes on in memory recall. This practitioner can support the person on the journey and, when the relevant memory source is reached, help him or her understand the connection between that past experience and present life and behavior patterns. Also, there may be a particular aroma that draws a person enigmatically to it, and there may be a story behind that.

I remember going to the Max Factor Museum in Los Angeles and being struck by an aroma I did not know. When I say "struck," I mean that inhaling it caused a profound reaction in my solar plexus. This aroma and I have a history, which I have yet to discover. It conjured up images of which I have no conscious memory, of a time before my birth. One day I'll return to that museum with my essential oil kit and attempt to replicate the aroma. Then, with the help of someone to guide me through the experience, I'll hopefully understand what significance it has for me.

If you have found while undergoing bodywork that you have memories, or any other experience that is different from normal, and there is an aroma attached to it that corresponds with an essential oil, take a sample of that next time you go and inhale it before the session begins. Ask the therapist to work on the same part that last time caused the memory or other reaction. Be very open with the therapist about this. It is important to verbalize any such experiences, and discuss them. Aside from the fact that you need to bring them into the open, so they can be released, if any event involved physical hurt, the energetic emotional reaction was probably stored in the body tissue and organs, and your therapist will want to know about it.

Whether there is an aroma memory or not, write down the details of any unusual happenings during bodywork sessions. Questions you might ask yourself are, Which part of the body was the therapist working on at the time? or What was the emotion I felt? Try to be conscious of what is occurring, as there may be important life lessons in it.

Reactions to particular aromas are highly individualistic. One that recalls a good memory in one person may bring a bad memory for another. One person may have no reaction at all, while another may find a far memory is revealed. Aromas are like pigments that color our experiences of life, and each painting is unique.

There have now been so many books, articles, and TV programs about past-life experiences, they can hardly be denied. The question is, What are they? In some cases, they are undoubtedly an illusion; someone has read something, overheard something, or seen something they later adopt as their own experience. In most cases, these are innocent mistakes, caused by being half-asleep, or in a daydream, or some mental state in which reality and fantasy become mixed up. Children may be particularly prone to this. If everything we ever see, smell, and hear is retained in our vast memory vault, who can say that a baby didn't watch a TV program in, say, 1960 and "recall" it as a "past life" in 2000? Some "past lives" might be pure hallucination, caused by mysterious events in the brain's biochemistry. Perhaps too, past lives are simply genetic memory, an invisible inheritance we carry deep within. Our parents' experiences might be our experiences, and we "inherit the sins of our fathers," as the Bible says, for seven generations. However, in many cases there is absolutely no possibility of this because the ancestors and the date and location of the recalled event don't match up. This is especially so in recalls relating to the past thirty years or so, when the whereabouts of ancestors can easily be confirmed.

Those who work in this field are familiar with the options, and are also familiar with the profound release that can come from experiencing key moments in past or far lives, and in the present life, and see that major changes in behavior and life direction can result. When a person is freed from encumbering emotions of the past or other lives, encountered along the spirit's journey, they soar like a bird into a happier future. This release can be physical, and chronic pains and ailments are sometimes said to lessen; it can be behavioral, and old ways of relating change for the better; and it can be spiritual, as people find their own true selves. In a sense it doesn't matter whether the techniques used access the personal subconscious or superconscious, or the universal consciousness. What is clear is that we find that which we seek and need to evolve. In this, aroma can play a transformational role.

Chapter 7

Fragrant Clouds of Purity and Protection

To wonder at nothing when it happens: to consider nothing impossible before it comes to pass.

— Cicero (106–43 BCE)

HUMAN BEINGS ARE FAR MORE SENSE-ATIVE than can be accounted for by sight, hearing, touch, taste, and smell. We react in different ways to people and places, "feeling" them to be beneficial to us or not, although such differences cannot be accounted for by the way they *look*. A person might walk into the room and appear perfectly normal, in that they are dressed like everyone else and behave in much the same way, but we might feel suddenly, unaccountably distressed. Or we might walk into a room and feel uncomfortable in it, though it's clean and well furnished. It may even be our own home that feels, at times, uncomfortable in a way we cannot explain.

Unseen energies are a part of life and, though invisible, affect us deeply and even change the course of our actions. People say, "I just want to get out of here," and although we may not have the same feeling, we understand that some unpleasant energy phenomenon has taken place, and reply, "Okay, let's go." You often hear people say of a person he or she "saps my energy." There's no energy to see, but we know exactly what they mean, and sympathize. You even hear people occasionally say, "I felt a presence in the room," and although we don't know exactly what this "presence" is, we've known similar experiences at some point in our lives, and accept what they say. Even though we may have a limited vocabulary to describe these invisible energy experiences, they are there nonetheless. If invisibility meant nonexistence, there would be no such thing as portable radios, televisions, and mobile telephones, because these are the receiving hardware that interpret bits of invisible information floating through the air. Our bodies are the receivers of other, natural, unseen energies, some of which are not welcome in our lives.

Judging by the number of age-old talismans, ceremonies, and rituals people use around the world, dealing with these unseen forces has been a very widespread human activity, with them being variously perceived as "bad luck," "the evil eye," "spirits," and in more modern times, "negative thought forms," "distressed emotional frequencies," and other similar terms. Some Christians wear a St. Christopher's medal as a pendant, to protect them while traveling, or the cross of the Crucifixion, while a feng shui expert might rearrange the furniture in a building to redirect the "wind and water" forces, to bring good energies and fortune.

When dealing with the invisible forces, and despite differences in belief, geographical location, and time, people have often used fragrance as a protective shield between them and the perceived negativity. This manipulation of fragrance for spiritual ends binds people very distant from each other in belief, space, and time, and often they use the same widely dispersed species of plant to facilitate more or less the same effect. Cedarwood, pine, and juniper are among those plants that have been widely adopted in this way.

Native Americans living along the Thompson River in British Columbia burned juniper to keep "ghosts" away, and in Tibet, juniper is offered daily to good spirits. In several Native American cultures, the aroma of burning sweetgrass or sage purifies the energies and attracts "supernaturals." In Arabic homes today, on Thursdays, frankincense is burned in a censer and carried through the living rooms and bedrooms to expel evil spirits and invite angels in. In the souk in Cairo, Egypt, people make a living going from shop to shop, censing each in turn with frankincense burned in a censer or even on a small piece of charcoal in a rusty tin can, to dispel any negative energy customers may have left behind, making the environment more inviting to potential customers.

Such practices have been going on for millennia. The ancient Mesopotamians, Egyptians, Greeks, and Romans all used fragrance not only to attract beneficial energy, but to keep inauspicious energies "at bay." The Greeks fumigated homes with bay leaves, while in the early days of Rome, verbena or other fragrant plants were hung above doorways to deter *il malocchio,* "the evil eye." Censers were kept burning by front doors in classical times, even by the poorer households. In medieval Europe, "witches" were the feared bad spirit, and rituals were carried out at pivotal points in the year with the object of dispelling them from the vicinity. These often involved walking through the village or town waving bunches of smoldering fragrant herbs or woods, to send the aroma into every nook and cranny. Juniper and rosemary were among those widely used. In the feng shui spirit-placating rite, *tun fu*, incense is used.

Many of the incense ingredients used throughout history and today are healing agents — myrrh, frankincense, cinnamon, clove, hyssop, sage, cedarwood, juniper, cypress, and pine, among others. No wonder then that incense and fragranced ointments and salves, which may well have conferred health, should be seen as "protective" — a beneficent agent of the deity, and this was especially the case when it was thought that physical health was inextricably linked to spiritual health.

The unfortunate Europeans who suffered during the plagues of the fourteenth to seventeenth centuries must have been sure they had in some way transgressed when they read this in the Old Testament: "If thou wilt diligently hearken to the voice of the Lord thy God, and wilt do that which is right in his sight, and wilt give ear to his commandments, and keep all his statutes, I will put none of these diseases upon thee, which I have brought upon the Egyptians: for I am the Lord that healeth thee." The agents for healing at this time, these people's saving grace, came in the form of fragrance and perfumers. Fragrant materials became highly sought after, especially rosemary, clove, garlic, rue, melissa, rose, lavender, and juniper, and were vital protection when in church for example. Around 1700, British author Daniel Defoe described one such scene in London: "The whole church was like a smelling bottle; in one corner it was all perfumes; in another aromatics, balsamics, and a variety of drugs and herbs; in another salts and spirits." In 1646 France, Arnaud Baric gave a full description of the role played by perfumers who, under the lead of "the health captain," passed through houses fumigating them with perfume burned on coal fires. At the end of the long day, the perfumers were themselves cleansed by standing in the "steaming room," a cloth tent with perfume material boiling away in a pot.

It is a curious thing that so many fragrant plants should be protective to the health. It is almost as if we are invited by the creative force of the universe to examine them, taste them, put them in our food, enjoy their aroma, and in other ways make use of them. The healing properties of many fragrant plants were of course well known in ancient times, which may account for the very widespread practice of aromatically cleansing strangers or guests before allowing them into the village or house.

A hundred years ago in central Borneo, the Blu-u Kayans burned bundles of fragrant plehiding bark when strangers arrived, to drive away any accompanying "evil spirits." In Turkey, Afghanistan, and Persia, visiting guests were first cleansed by burning branches of fragrant plants or incense, while aboriginal Australians saved their hosts the trouble and came with their own lighted bark or fragrant burning sticks. As well as fragrance, fire and loud noise have been widely employed, as author J. G. Frazer states in *The Golden Bough*, "for the purpose of disarming the strangers of their magical powers, of counteracting the baneful influence which is believed to emanate from them, or of disinfecting, so to speak, the tainted atmosphere by which they are supposed to be surrounded." In the contemporary world, the practice of aromatic cleansing is still ubiquitous in the Middle East, where it is perceived as a hospitable kindness to guests. In tents in the desert a few small pieces of aromatic resin may be put on the brazier, while in towns visitors are more likely to be greeted with rose water sprinkled from a long-stemmed *gulabdan*. Guests in Turkish households have lemon-scented cologne sprinkled on the hands, so it can be wiped on the arms and neck. This fragrant nicety is also offered by the conductor to passengers on long-distance buses.

Fragrance is also widely used to cleanse buildings, especially those used for spiritual practices. When Saladin retook the Mosque of Omar at Jerusalem from the Christians in 1187 CE, he had it purified with rose water; and when Mohamet II captured the Church of Sancta Sophia in Constantinople in 1453 CE, and made it a mosque, it was likewise first treated with rose. Sage is the most sacred herb of the Yuwipe Native American nation, and it is this that covers the floor of the medicine man's house, as he goes about the purification process.

Fragrance and spirituality have always been inextricably linked. In Mesopotamia four thousand years ago, incense was used both to attract the goddesses and gods, and to repel malevolent spirits. In Muslim terminology, jinni are said to be an order of spirits that can assume human and animal form and exercise negative influence over people, and *pirs* are people brought in to deal with them — often incorporating the inhalation of jasmine oil as part of the proceedings.

THE BENEFICENT HOME

Our home should be an oasis of peace, or at least a place where we feel at home with ourselves — centered and complete, healthy, creative, and joyful. Most of the time this may be the case, but if we've been burglarized, the house just feels "dirty" — even, as one person told me, when a cat burglar silently went through her place wearing thick gloves and disturbing nothing but the safe. The initial reaction after such a violation is often, "It doesn't feel like it's my place anymore; I want to move *now*," but this is seldom a practical possibility. If we move home, to a place previously occupied by other people, again, the energies can feel "not right."

It is not only the energy of those who are present that we have to think about, but the energy of those who have passed through that particular space before. Walls, so it is said, hold the energy of people who occupied that room in former times. The love and joy, or fear, anger, and pain, somehow get imprinted in the very fabric of the building. Whether this is the case or not, it is certainly true that walls hold ancient aromas, as has been discovered by commercial dehumidifier workers who smell the aroma of incense burned long ago emanating from the walls of churches during treatment. Aroma is a tangible thing, compared with love, fear, and thought, but all have a vibration and an energy that can linger.

Healers who work within the auric fields of people — the energy field around the body of a person — feel that field, in some cases, as sticky. This same gray etheric-quagmire sort of quality can suffuse a home, or a room in it, and can be felt by sensitive people and animals. It's variously described as "thick," "heavy," and "dim."

After a burglary, or when moving into a new place, it's very appropriate that we perform a spiritual cleansing, but even invited visitors to our home can often leave their vibrational imprint behind. If those people are full of sadness or misery, or are the kind of people who radiate negativity or soak up positivity, that can be a real burden on the energy of the premises (as well as on us!). They leave feeling replenished, but you and the house feel depleted — and it may be time to work on the energy of both you and the place.

When a building holds energies that have a detrimental effect, they can be expressed as, perhaps, the feeling that the place is never really clean (despite the fact that, to look at and touch, it is clean); and often the inhabitant wants to clean it over and over again. Conversely, there may be the feeling that you don't want to clean, touch, or disturb anything; a general feeling of discomfiture; a desire to always rearrange furniture; or, simply, being depressed as soon as you open the front door. The energies in a home can also account for physical sensations: feeling tired all the time, getting headaches, or feeling pressure on the head. Clearly, these things could also be symptoms of some physical disorder, and before considering the energetic quality of a home as the cause, see your doctor for a checkup. Obviously, too, if there have been arguments in a home, they may account for an atmosphere of disquiet; and electromagnetic fields generated by electrical pylons, for example, have been said to account for the symptoms listed above.

CLEARING THE ATMOSPHERE

Rooms can have a different atmosphere that cannot always be attributed to such things as decor, lighting, ceiling height, or even good or bad feng shui — there's the flow of *chi*, or life energy, around a home, which depends on its location and the placement of doors, windows, furniture, mirrors, and plants, among other things. Rooms also have an aroma that reflects all that is in, and goes on, there, including activities such as cooking; the aroma of things such as furnishings; and the presence of living beings such as people, animals, and plants. Humidity can change an atmosphere, and the aroma of mildew can these days be treated with various commercial products and appliances, while the dryness of central heating can be counterbalanced with humidifiers. Bear all these things in mind when considering the atmosphere of a room or home.

Another factor is cleanliness. If a place does not feel conducive to good energy flow, it may simply need a good clean. We're not talking here about untidiness, but uncleanness, the solution to which is obvious. When thinking about cleaning in terms of energy, however, add salt to the water, along with some essential oils, whatever aroma you enjoy.

As you go around your home, take a box and throw in all those items of clutter that you know you will no longer use, or you don't really like. According to the philosophy of feng shui, they clutter your mind, as well as your home, and could be given to a charity shop, which may benefit from them more than you. Washing windows is especially good for energy flow. It gives a different look to the outside of a home, and a different feel to the inside. Add essential oils to either the water or to the cloth — the citrus oils are particularly good for this job.

Spiritual cleansing is different to the usual cleaning routine and involves much more thought, and a little more preparation. Here is a traditional method of transforming the subtle energies of a room. Before you start, focus your mind on the job at hand, and invoke that which is the source of your spiritual strength. Pray that the cleansing will bring light and peace. Mix a tablespoon of salt with two drops of frankincense essential oil, and leave it to dry. Open a window or a door leading to the outside, which allows circulation of air, then sprinkle a tiny amount of the mixture around the room, including the corners, gradually moving toward the open window or door.

Another method involves using salt water in a bowl, wetting the fingers and flicking the water in all directions, being careful not to damage certain fabrics and furniture. Essential oils can be added to this water-salt mix. A very ancient method is to dip a small bundle of fresh herbs into salt water, shake off the excess, and use this to flick the water around the room. Some cultures use a small branch of a tree; you could also use a single flower.

The spiritual house-cleansing process can be done while diffusing your favorite essential oils. Some people pray while cleansing; others use loud noise, which has often been used to scare negative elements away. This can be done in the traditional way, with drums, bells, rattles, gongs, clapping, or chanting, although I know people who prefer loud music, as they feel this is very effective in getting the energy up and moving. When the atmosphere feels lightened, use one of the following cleansing blends of essential oils, or an essential oil or blend of your choice — in a diffuser, plant mister, or simply in a bowl or mug of steaming water. Put on some tranquil music, light a candle, then have a cleansing bath — suggestions for which are in a later section. Finally, put some new life and happiness in the room or rooms in the form of plants or flowers.

CLEANSING BLENDS *for Diffusers, Herb Bundles, Misters, and Water Bowls*					
Frankincense	7 drops	Pine	5 drops	Lemon	3 drops
Benzoin	2 drops	Fir	3 drops	Orange	3 drops
Myrrh	1 drop	Cypress	2 drops	Grapefruit	4 drops
Sage	2 drops	Sage	2 drops	Clove	3 drops
Cedar	6 drops	Myrtle	6 drops	Black Pepper	3 drops
Juniper	2 drops	Hyssop	2 drops	Cinnamon	4 drops
Coriander	5 drops	Rose	6 drops	Spikenard	3 drops
Fennel	2 drops	Jasmine	2 drops	Ginger	4 drops
Dill	2 drops	Linden Blossom	2 drops	Vetiver	3 drops

Misters and Sprayers

One effective method of distributing the essential oil molecules around a space is by using a plant mister or sprayer. Using a new one, put in half a pint of warm water, then add six to ten drops of essential oil — or more if you wish — screw back the cap, and shake well each time before spraying. Spray high into the air, making sure the water–essential oil molecules will not fall on any furniture or furnishings that may become damaged. The space around people can also be sprayed with these "aura cleansing sprays," but the eyes must be kept closed.

Water Bowls

Hot water releases the aroma molecules in essential oils and sends them rising into the air. Any glass or china heatproof bowl or container can be used. Put three to ten drops of essential oil on the water, and place the bowl or bowls in the corners of the room.

Essential Oil Cleansing Bundles

Make a collection of smelling strips by cutting up a piece of white absorbent paper into long strips. Put your chosen essential oils on these. They can be gathered together like a bunch of flowers, and tied with bows, or plaited, and in other ways made decorative. Use them to spread cleansing- and energy-enhancing fragrance around a room.

Using Salt for Spiritual Cleansing

There are many ways to use salt as part of spiritual cleansing. It can be used on its own or mixed with essential oils. It can be put in water and used to purify rooms, spaces, objects, and people. It can be added to baths.

Essential oils can be added to salt and crushed minerals or gems, such as crystals, and used to purify rooms and objects, or put in baths. Which particular essential oils, gems, or salt you use will depend on what you are setting out to achieve.

As the seas are so polluted these days, sea salt may carry those vibrations, but it also carries the energy of the sea. Rock salt gives the energy of the mountains and the earth.

ENERGY-CLEANSING BATHS

Every time we walk into an enclosed space, whether it is at work, on the bus, in a shop, cinema, or theater, we are putting ourselves in contact with other people's electromagnetic fields. Our auras mingle, for example, when standing shoulder to shoulder with other commuters in an underground train during rush hour. Some of these people may be disturbed, distressed, or depressed and in other ways energetically needy. The interaction of energies between people involves a give-and-take. There is the good giving, when we feel enriched energetically, and there is the kind of giving that comes from a very "hyper" person, which leaves one feeling exhausted. With taking, the issue is a willingness to donate that energy. We don't mind giving energy to our children, for example, and we freely allow the people we love to take energy from us, even though it may leave us feeling depleted. But there is also the kind of taking when people draw the energy out of us, a kind of energetic violation, although most energy vampires may not consciously be aware of what they're doing. I've found that many of these people have been energetically abused at some time in the past and have an unstable personal boundary.

This is not just a physical-presence phenomenon, because we can find ourselves giving and taking in relation to another person, even over the phone. In fact, we don't even need that equipment, because we can hear the phone ringing on the other side of the room and know from the change in our energy that on the end of the line is a specific someone we don't want to talk to. When they say their name, they just confirm what we had already sensed in some inexplicable way.

The effect of all this can be disturbing to our own vibrational pattern, and there may be times when we feel the need of a spiritually cleansing bath. The purpose of this is to "wash off" the unwanted thought forms or energies we may have picked up. Spiritual cleansing is about preserving the integrity of our spiritual core. It is of particularly great importance when we've had the unfortunate experience of being in touch — which may not be literal — with a person whose vibration is altogether nefarious.

Energy-cleansing baths are not about removing everyday grime and pollution, which should be done first by having a shower or bath and washing with soap. First, clear and enhance the atmosphere by using one of the methods in the Clearing the Atmosphere or Holy Smoke — for Purification sections in this chapter. Open the window or door to oxygenate the room. Some of the old traditions would use sound at this point, with clapping, chanting, drumbeating, singing, praying, laughing, shaking rattles, or shouting, and if your inclination is to use sound, you could use one of those methods, or check through your music collection for something that seems appropriate.

For people who want to bring in the four elements of water, earth, fire, and air, these are already present. The water flows into the bath; the earth comes from the salt or crystals you place in the water; the fire comes from the candles you now place around the bath; and the air comes from the fresh air you have just allowed in the room and the aroma of the essential oils you will use.

Essential oils on their own are rather unique among the gifts of life in that they incorporate in some sense all four elements — they are liquid and thus waterlike; they are products of plants of the earth; they are flammable and burn like fire; and they release a fragrance that is part of the air.

Bathing or being submerged in water is a sacred symbolic ritual in many traditions, often signifying full entry into a particular practice or way of worship. It also symbolizes rebirth and change, whether this is a change in the direction of life or in its purpose. Cleaning invisible energies with water is an everyday occurrence at nuclear power stations around the world, as workers finish their shift with a shower to assist in removing any radiation. Bathing is about being "clean" in many senses.

Focus on what you wish to achieve from your bath, and review the essential oil spiritual profiles in chapter 11 to choose those that seem particularly useful at this time. Essential oils carry the energy of the original flower or plant, yet have undergone transformation through fire and water in the distillation process. Again, all four elements are present: in the earth of the plant material, the fire that lights the still, and the water that extracts the essential oil molecules, which are then released into the air. The essential oils help cleanse the energetic field of the water, whether you use single essential oils, make your own blends, or try one of those suggested below.

ENERGY-CLEANSING BATH BLENDS

Add up to two tablespoons of salt to the flowing water. When the bath has been run, add the essential oils, swishing them around a bit, with a prayer in your heart. These blends can also be used in diffusers, herb bundles, misters, water bowls, or essential oil cleansing bundles.

Neroli	3 drops	Myrtle	3 drops	Rosemary	2 drops
Orange	1 drop	Clary Sage	1 drop	Eucalyptus	1 drop
Petitgrain	2 drops	Lemon	1 drop	Lavender	3 drops
Chamomile	3 drops	Frankincense	4 drops	Rose	3 drops
Mandarin	3 drops	Lemon	2 drops	Neroli	3 drops

THE ELEMENTS

When carrying out purification, you may want to incorporate all the elements or only those you consider essential. Some traditions, for example, include wood or metal among the core elements; others do not. What you use is a matter of personal choice as you devise what suits you at any particular time.

When cleansing a room or person with essential oils or herb bundles, focus on the four directions in turn — north, south, east, and west — and carry the fragrant material in those directions before making a complete circle. In some cultures, before doing the circle, the fragrant material would be lowered to the earth and then raised to the sky.

The following chart shows some of the ways people bring the elements into purification and cleansing practices:

USING THE ELEMENTS FOR PURIFICATION AND CLEANSING							
Fire	*Air*	*Earth*	*Water*	*Sound*	*Metal*	*Wood*	*Light*
Candles	Aroma	Salt	Bowls	Prayer	Gold	Sticks	Candles
Diffusers	Open windows	Stones	Misters/ Sprays	Chanting	Silver	Wooden objects	Mirrors
Incense	Open doors	Crystals	Fountains	Singing	Copper	Incense	Open curtains to let the sun in
Open curtains to let the sun in	Wind chimes	Flowers		Music			
		Plants		Mantras			
Fireplace	Plants	Herbs					
		Fruit peel					

HOLY SMOKE — FOR PURIFICATION

Smoke comes from fire, always considered one of the main elements in purification, along with prayer. Obviously one cannot burn that which one wishes to purify, as there'd be nothing left! So, the best thing to use is smoke. In Buddhist temples in Japan and China, the smoke from burning material is used not only to send prayers upward, but to smoke the body for spiritual cleansing, purification, and healing of the auric field. People can be seen using their cupped hands to direct the smoke over their heads and shoulders before entering the temple. Incense is often used, and as I have discovered on occasion, some rather less aromatically pleasing materials. I have found myself in thick, pungent clouds of smoke, which filled my lungs and hung to my clothes all day.

The small lumps of resinous incense burned in censers in Christian churches, particularly of the Orthodox and Coptic traditions, can produce large amounts of smoke, which not only pervade the building but engulf the congregation within. Native Americans use "smudge sticks" made of fragrant herbs, grasses, and leaves from trees, directing the smoke with a feather around people as well as places.

All these and other traditions use the smoke of natural, fragrant plant materials. The purpose of these ceremonies may be specific in that they mark a rite of passage such as birth, menarche, manhood, marriage, menopause, retirement, and death, or aim to improve ill health. They may be more general in that they aim to cleanse the auric field and alter the energy residing within a space or emanating from a person. Smoking is thought to clear negative influences, restore balance, induce spiritual purification, increase spiritual awareness, and prepare the mind-body-spirit for sacred ceremony. Smoke is also used to cleanse environments, whether at home or work, and in exorcism.

Essential oils incorporate the two elements that constitute the smoke ceremonies — fire and fragrant plant material. They do not of themselves produce smoke, unless burned on charcoal, but many people find this to be an advantage. In burning fragrant plant material, the aroma is released by the heat, but so too is a great deal of smoke. Essential oils are also readily available, whereas some of the plant materials traditionally used are not. Essential oils can be used on their own, in diffusers or simply on smelling strips, and directed as in smoke ceremonies around the head and body of a person, or around a room.

Whatever material is used, and whatever the purpose, the other crucial element is spiritual thought. As you go about the business of using holy smoke, or essential oils on their own, invoke your spiritual source and put your whole mind into asking for assistance in achieving your goal.

Essential oils are flammable, and care should be taken with them when using fire of any kind. The only time I recommend using essential oils in conjunction with fire is in candles, by the method described in chapter 2. Shop-bought "aromatherapy" candles may contain synthetic fragrances, which have nothing to do with aromatherapy or cleansing and purification. You can make your own essential oil candles using candle-making kits and pure, natural essential oils.

Natural resins have, of course, been placed on braziers or censers for millennia, but few of us own the equipment to replicate this system of use. If you do, the incenses traditionally used, depending on the culture, include frankincense, myrrh, copal, benzoin, and gum arabic in resin form. In Asia, especially Japan, fragrant woods such as jinko, kara-mokkoh, and kyara are highly prized and come in delicate strips that are placed on charcoal or in small incense burners. They are generally used to raise the spiritual energetic level of a person, rather than for purification and protection.

If you have a fireproof incense dish, usually made of pottery or metal, essential oils can be used in conjunction with small round pieces of charcoal that are sold specifically for use with incense. But, be warned, the effect is dramatic as the essential oil smoke shoots high into the air, and before trying this method you should do a test-run outside and stand well back. The charcoal does not always look as if it's alight when it actually is, so care must be taken. Patience is required, as the charcoal will light in one place and tiny sparks can be seen running across the surface as the heat activates the entire piece, which can still at this point be black. In fact, it is red-hot without the red color! Wait until this process is complete before adding the essential oils in moderation.

Fragrant Plant Bundles

In the Native American spiritual traditions, smudging plays a central role. Smudge sticks are long bundles of fragrant plant material, wound tight, lit at one end until the material catches fire, then blown out so it continues to smolder, releasing the smoke.

The fragrant materials used by Native Americans are usually sage, wormwood, cedar, or sweetgrass. Occasionally, depending on the location within the United States and Canada, the soft young stems of pine are used. These have pine needles attached and are very pliable. There is also a plant called "prairie lavender" that is included in the smudge sticks of certain nations, which is not of the same species of lavender known throughout Europe but somehow acquired the name from early European settlers.

Sage

There are many types of sage, including *Salvia apiana*, which can grow very tall and live for more than one hundred years. Another variety often used is *Salvia columbarne*. Sagebrush, *Artemisia tridentata*, belongs to the wormwood family rather than to the sage.

Wormwood

Artemisias belong to the wormwood family, although they are sometimes called sage. They bear no resemblance to the sages known in Europe. In Native American culture, *Artemisia spinescens* is sometimes used in smudge sticks.

Cedar

Often the trees that are called cedar are actually of the juniper family, such as *Juniperus virginiana*. All types of cedar needles are also used, including *Thuya occidentalis*.

Sweetgrass

This is sometimes called vanilla grass, and is *Hierochloe odorata,* a tall green grass that becomes yellowish when dried. On drying, its aroma becomes more apparent. In some nations it is put on the hot stones of sweat lodges.

In these processes, it is the leaves and soft stalks of the plant that are used. Smudge sticks are held in the hand, carrying the smoke to where it's required, or the smoke is directed by the hands or with a feather. Other cultures use a small branch of a plant or tree to direct the smoke, often of the same species as that used in the smoldering fragrant material. You could also use big crystals to spread the smoke around, or other stones that you are attuned to, or amber, which is a resin from a plant.

Making Your Own Smudge Sticks or Herb Bundles

Before starting any activity as spiritually directed as making herb bundles, wash yourself, or at the very least wash your hands and forearms, letting the water run down them. This flushes away any energy held.

All plants that are picked and dried should be honored. Take only one stem or two so the plant can continue to flourish. Have empathy, and show the plant respect. Ask permission of the plant, that you may take this branch to perform your spiritual practice. Your intuition will tell you whether it is right or wrong — when another plant should be chosen.

Pick stems that are long enough to be bound together. Look in your garden to see what has grown and matured. The herb garden is a good place to start, and you could use sage, lavender, rosemary, thyme, oregano, or clary sage. If you have access to cypress or pine, you could use a small young branch. It is sometimes said that herbs or other material that are indigenous to the region should be used, but my favorite, Californian white sage, comes from a place far from my home.

Arrange the stems and leaves, not using so much that there will be difficulty in burning, or too much smoke produced. Put the stems in an elastic band, which will keep the pieces together while you tie the bundle, and remove it when you've finished. Take a long piece of cotton thread, doubled, and place the top of the bundle in the middle. Using the two ends, bind the bundle together tightly, in a crisscross fashion. Start at the top, crisscrossing the length of the bundle, and finish by winding the cotton around the bottom part of the stems. You'll now have a cone-shaped bundle. It needs to dry before it'll burn, so hang it upside down in a dry place — an airing cabinet would be ideal.

Essential oils can be added to your bundle before tying. They are highly concentrated energy forms and will increase the energetic potential of the plants. Use them in moderation; remember they are flammable. Try to use an essential oil or oils that are compatible with your bundle, being from the same kind of plant. However, if a particular herb, plant, or tree — such as cypress, cedar, or pine — is not available, by adding that essential oil, of pine for example, you can bring that energy into the smoke.

To use the herb bundle, ignite the end, then put out the fire so it's just smoldering. Hold a small fireproof bowl under the bundle to catch any lit pieces that may drop as the bundle burns. Then walk around the room slowly, wafting the smoke into all the corners so it gradually clears away negative influences and energizes the protective, cleansing frequencies. If smudging a person, walk around them; if smudging yourself, move the bundle around yourself, or move your body, so the smoke can enfold you. Start around the top, moving down to the feet, where the energy will disperse into the ground. The smoke can be directed with a cupped hand, a feather, a bunch of fresh herbs or leaves, a flower, or mineral, whatever feels right to you.

Do this with pure thought. Some people do it with prayer, chanting, or singing. When you have finished, place the bundle down carefully with a fireproof dish underneath, as it might still contain burning material. Then open a window.

Decorative Bundles

If you do not plan to burn the bundle, a whole world of possibilities open up. Bundles can be bound incorporating color, texture, and meaning. Essential oils will add fragrance and energy. Try flowers like marigold or rose. Spices such as cinnamon sticks and clove, and fruits in the form of dried lemon or orange peel, are cleansing in their own right. Small pieces of fragrant wood can be added and depending on how you plan to display the bundle, other objects wound into the arrangement, such as crystals and minerals, and the small light rocks that are the resins in their original form.

Herbal Smoke Bowls

Another method of using smoke involves putting a drop of an essential oil on a small amount of dried material, on a big shell or a piece of fireproof pottery or glass, then setting light to the material, putting out the flame to release the smoke.

Chapter 8

Multidimensional Bodies

*Just as the body is composed of various things and is nourished by
various foods so the spirit is likewise composed of, and enjoys and is
nourished by, a certain variety of air. The spirit must be daily refreshed
by this kind of variety, for air and odor seem almost like spirits. . . .*
— Marsilio Ficino, b. 1433, "On Air and Odors,"
from *The Book of Life*

THERE WILL ALWAYS BE MYSTERIES — the universe is too large for anything but that. I'm hoping, though, that in the not too distant future science will be able to explain one of the most intriguing aspects of life, multidimensional radiant bodies. Aside from the physical body, we have an "aura," a light that surrounds the body and is often depicted as a halo in paintings of saints and holy people. We also have energy centers in the body known as "chakras" and some say an "etheric body," an "astral body," and a "mental body," all usually invisible energy fields that connect us to the universe. These names have arisen from the European esoteric tradition of the early twentieth century, which has its roots in ancient Indian and other Asian philosophies. More recently, people talk in terms of the "light body," the "emotional body," and the "auric field," all of which are aspects of the same phenomenon.

Very few people can see auras or chakras, let alone the etheric, astral, or mental bodies. This is not to say they don't exist. Anyone with the right kind of sensitivity, opportunity, and practice could, if doing regular therapeutic work with people, feel the auric field and chakras. Many of us might have an idea of the way the various energy fields, or "bodies," might be operating, but in this area of study there is a great deal of speculation and little scientific proof.

One person who has done valuable work in this area is scientist Dr. Valerie Hunt, working both with the most technologically advanced equipment and specialist research environments, and with people with visionary powers that are as ancient, probably, as the human race itself. Some people would call what she studies "the aura," although Dr. Hunt, author of *The Infinite Mind: The Science of Human Vibrations*, prefers the term "energy field." At the same time as machinery recorded electromagnetic energy in people subjected to various research procedures, clairvoyants and healers recorded what they saw. The correlation between these, taken together with the concurrent recorded experiences of the research participants, including herself, led Dr. Hunt to hypothesize that "the energy field is the highest level of the mind of man, and that it is through this level that we interrelate with the cosmosphere."

It's well known that there's an alternating electrical system that can be measured with electrodes placed on the surface of the body. This alternating current of the nervous system affects a great deal including the brain, muscles, glands, and our touch sensation. The on-off quality of this energy is reflected in the beat of a heart, the contract-relax double action of a muscle, and the peaks and dips of a brain wave. Many of us have had this energy monitored through, for example, an electrocardiograph (ECG) machine, which measures electrical heart function, or an electroencephalograph (EEG) machine, which measures the electrical activity from different parts of the brain.

Dr. Hunt was interested in another form of electromagnetic energy in the body, which is thought to derive from the fact that each subatomic particle and cell in the body has an electrical element. She discovered that this second energy is continuous, not alternating. From her recordings, the data that related to brain, heart, and muscle frequencies (0 to 250 cycles per second) could be removed to identify data coming from this second electromagnetic system (which oscillates at 500 to 20,000 cycles per second, and maybe more as the machinery couldn't record any higher). This energy field is smaller in amplitude and higher in frequency than the brain-heart-muscle system, and eight to ten times faster. The millivoltage is between a half and a third as strong as that of a resting muscle. Changes in readings from this energy field, caused by sound or light, occurred before those in the body. Dr. Hunt believes "a person's primary response in this world takes place first in the auric field, not in the sensory nerves nor in the brain." The field apparently increases when a person walks barefoot on grass, or takes a swim or a cold shower, "probably because of the increased negative ions," says Dr. Hunt.

At the physics department of the University of California in Los Angeles, the research continued in the Mu room — a seven-foot-square environment in which the electromagnetic energy of the air can be manipulated. It's large enough to accommodate more than one person, adding an extra dimension to the experiments. There Dr. Hunt discovered that if the electrical level was reduced, the "aura" or "energy field" became disorganized and the subjects lost the sense of where their bodies were located in the space. When the electromagnetism was depleted, there was more interaction between the fields of the people as each would try to compensate by drawing on the energy of another in the room. The result was everyone's field became even more depleted.

All of this is fascinating enough, but there were more interesting effects to discover. If the electrical field in the room was increased, the auric fields returned to their usual state and the people reported an expansion of consciousness and clarity of thought. When the electrical level in the room was normal, but the magnetism decreased, the people found simple coordination tests, such as putting a finger to the nose, difficult. With the electricity the same, but the magnetism increased, the subjects had vastly increased motor ability, being able to lean over at an extraordinary angle and to balance on the toes of one foot.

Working concurrently with clairvoyants, Dr. Hunt discovered that when the auric field was depleted in the Mu room, a fishnet effect of energy could be seen flowing through the whole body. The pattern of the flow did not correspond with the meridian lines of classical Chinese medicine, for example, but seemed more to follow the path of connective tissue.

Dr. Hunt also carried out research involving rolfers, therapists who deeply manipulate the connective tissue of the body. Such manipulation can cause a person to feel emotional, see pictures in the mind, and remember incidents from the past. It was found that if a subject experienced imagery, spontaneous pictures, there was a back-and-forth energy shift between the throat and brow chakras. Memory appears to be related to chakra, or energy-center, activity.

Many other eminent scientists have tried to measure the electromagnetic field, starting with Karl von Reichenbach, who called it an "odic force"; Harold Burr, who in *Blueprint for Immortality* spoke of "life fields"; Vladimir Inyushin, who referred to "bioplasma"; and Robert Becker, author of *The Body Electric*, among others. There have also been those who have captured the energy in photographic form, notably Semyon and Valentina Kirlian. Many of the electromagnetic researchers worked in relative obscurity but today, on many a main street, you can have your aura visually recorded by "aura imaging" or Kirlian photography cameras.

THE SUBTLE BODIES

Theosophical literature states that there are three bodies aside from the physical. They are presented here not as fact but as a sounding board or framework we can use to think more deeply about the subject of multidimensional bodies.

The Etheric Body, or "The Body of Light"

- This body is the blueprint upon which the physical body is built; the densest of the subtle bodies.

- This body is a field of energy that exists within the same space as the physical body, and interpenetrates it.

- The field is composed of many threads of energy, with light and force; the body of light.

- As in a web, it connects us to all parts of the universe; it connects us to higher realms.

- It vitalizes the physical body.

- It has a threefold action:
  - It receives energy.
  - It assimilates energy.
  - It transmits energy.

- The threads of energy crisscross through our etheric body, and energy centers, or chakras, occur where many lines cross. There are thought to be seven main chakras, five along the line of the spine and two in the head, plus many minor chakras.

The Mental Body

- This body is an ovoid mist that encloses all other bodies. It has very fine colors.

- It is very much affected by everything in our environment.

- It interacts strongly with astral matter.

- We control the fineness or the density of our mental body by the quality of our thoughts; spiritual thoughts produce higher vibrations.

The Astral Body, or "Emotional Body"

- There are seven subplanes of astral matter that, in different proportions and density, form a parallel world to the physical, which it interpenetrates; each type of physical matter attracts astral matter of the same density.

- It is composed of very fine substance, constantly moving; with colors.

- This body is where the feelings, emotions, and passions are expressed; it acts as a bridge between the physical brain and the "mind."

- When a person dies, his or her consciousness withdraws into the astral body and continues its journey on the astral plane. A living person can "leave their body" temporarily and go "astral traveling."

- The aura is the manifestation of the astral body and extends from the surface of the physical body to varying degrees, from a few inches to feet, or yards, or farther. The aura can be seen as color, and felt.

Auras are an aspect of our natural selves and the natural world. There is nothing weird or magical about them. Some people can see and feel them, while others can't, and this has less to do with any special powers of perception than with our desire to experience them and our application to that goal. Here then are some ways to expand your vision and sense of touch.

The first exercise involves trying to see a phenomenon that Austrian psychoanalyst Wilhelm Reich called "orgone dots" and theosophical literature calls "vitality globules." One of the best descriptions came from Jirij Moskvitin in *Essay on the Origin of Thought*, wherein he talks about brilliant sparks of dancing light, describing them as having tiny "tails." These light particles dart through the atmosphere in all directions, and the easiest way to see them is in daylight, against a light blue sky.

To see them, another method of looking is required, as with "magic eye" pictures, which appear at first like a disorganized but repetitive pattern of color. To see these pictures, the eyes are crossed or made to focus differently; to see the shimmering light particles, you need to get beyond normal vision, not by going cross-eyed, but instead by focusing in the distance, as if you were looking for a

To Feel Your Own Aura

First, with both hands opposite each other move the hands quickly in a repeated chopping movement, with one hand going down while the other goes up (body therapists know this movement as "hacking"), keeping your hands about four inches apart in the air in front of you. Then run a hand up your arm, about three inches away. It will be easier now to feel the electrical pull.

To See Your Own Aura

Carry out the chopping movement described in To Feel Your Own Aura, then place a hand over a piece of white or light-colored paper. In the right light you may be able to see your aura as a thin layer of light. When we connect with things, as when picking them up, the aura of the body extends to enfold the object, so the white line will be seen not only around the fingers, but also the pen or whatever we touch that has been brought into the field.

You can play with this energy field, moving the object slowly and watching the auric field enlarge and soften as it drags behind. I've watched this interaction with the human energy field using leaves, flowers, and, of course, essential oils. This phenomenon raises all kinds of questions, but it may explain why some people "get along" with some machines and some don't: perhaps the electromagnetic energy field of people differs enough to have different effects on machines.

Perhaps, too, it goes some way toward explaining how psychometrists work. These are sensitives, or clairvoyants, who can hold a piece of jewelry or an object belonging to another person and "read" it, by relating the emotions and circumstances of the person it belongs to. They may be tapping into the energy field that still lingers from the owner, a field that, if it can store information, must be rather "intelligent."

Aura Fluffing

Agitating the aura makes it become clearer and lighter. This is a kind of auric maintenance, as if dusting it off. The movement is a fluffing or flapping of the hands, moving them vigorously in the area five or six inches above the surface of the body.

Aura fluffing may have been what some of the ancient traditions did when "working" in this area, such as when Native Americans fan or wave a feather in the auric field, as part of a smoke ritual, including the use of smudge sticks; or when African shamans wave a bunch of herbs or a rattle near the body of a person.

One interesting aspect of aura fluffing is that it can reveal "referred pain syndrome"; that is, when pain appears in one part of the body although it has its source in another. If the aura is fluffed, for example, around an area of burning pain in the shoulder and neck, that pain may relocate (or appear to relocate) as a contraction in a muscle under the scapula (the shoulder blade). When the true original site of any problem can be located, a more accurate treatment can be applied to it.

Aura fluffing briefly dissipates the density of the aura, allowing it to rebalance itself, cleansed and energized.

spaceship in the far blue yonder. The first thing you may see are little gray or see-through wiggly pieces, which are on the surface of the eye and are probably some kind of dust. Then, going beyond them, some people see a watery effect, as if watching water running downward in a wave pattern on a piece of glass. Going beyond that, you begin to see small dancing flashes of light that seem to flicker on and off but that can be followed and seen to be individual-ized particles continuing a vitalized course. These globules appear like gold or silver, which could be the light reflecting off them, and some have very light translucent colors. They can be seen even from an aircraft window, and at that altitude they appear to be larger and clearer. Once you have seen light globules it becomes much easier to understand that the atmosphere is full of energy, and actually quite dense.

If you spray essential oils into the air, the light globules are attracted to the aroma molecules, and combine with them. To try this yourself, don't use the usual spray/misting method, which involves water, but instead use a small perfume sprayer and pure undiluted essential oils. Watching the attraction of aroma molecules and dancing light is an interesting experience, and makes me wonder what relationship they have. There is certainly a great deal yet to learn. Intriguingly, the French National Center for Scientific Research, in conjunction with the National Center for Space Studies, in France, has carried out research that shows, according to author Annick Le Guerer in *Scent*, "aromatic molecules are one of the basic components of the interstellar space in which new stars are constantly being formed. This interstellar 'atmosphere' or gas is also the almost-direct source of the atoms of which we ourselves, along with the earth and the other planets, are made."

ESSENTIAL OILS AND THE HUMAN AURIC FIELD

Having worked with essential oils in therapeutic practice for so many years, and having seen how they can affect the human aura, it was a great pleasure to watch their dynamic interactions through polycontrast interface photography (PIP), invented by Harry Oldfield, coauthor of *The Dark Side of the Brain*. As well as taking images of the energy field of essential oils on the end of a smelling strip, a few of which are shown on pages 125–28, we watched the essential oils interacting with the head, or hand and arm, or whole body. The energy of the essential oil radiates outward from the drop of that oil, touching upon the human · aura and enlivening it.

The photographs reproduced in this section show the effect when a drop of essential oil is placed in the palm of the hand, and the auric field is seen to be far more vibrant, colorful, and wider than in the control situation, when the subject is photographed with no essential oil.

Essential oils are a way of connecting cosmic energy to us. Plants take the energy of the sun and transform it, through photosynthesis, into the food energy upon which all animals rely. Essential oils are the concentrated form of that sun energy, and as can be seen from their auric pictures, highly energetic. Their vibrations can, by close association and harmonic vibration, transfer to us the ultimate source of that energy, cosmic power.

Using essential oils in the auric field brings a new energy to the field. The colors of the aura become brighter and clearer, while a shift in the density of the aura, and the energy above the chakras, can be felt. If the vibration of a

person is low for any reason, from a depressed mental state or ill health, the essential oils can stir or agitate the auric field, stimulating it to reorganize itself into a state of harmony. The simple way to look at this is to say it "lifts" the spirit by raising the vibration. But it is not the essential oil itself that causes the lift in spirit, it is the human organism with the aid of the oils. The essential oils do, however, clear the auric quagmire in which we may have got stuck, allowing us freedom to shift our perspective, change our spiritual position, and move on to a higher state of being.

Picture a television screen that is "out of sync." The colors have not all put themselves in the right — the same — location, and there's a shadow around the images. By adjusting the antenna, we bring the images back into sync, the same place, locked together in the proper position so a coherent whole results. Essential oils seem to have the same effect on the human aura, or bodies, bringing them into sync, locked together in a harmonious whole. Harmonized in this way, we are better able to get in touch with our higher selves, our spiritual core, the source of our strength.

Choosing Essential Oils for Subtle Energy Work

There is a flow of energy, not only between essential oils and people, but between people and essential oils. It's a two-way street. When choosing essential oils at any time, then, we need to consider the source of those oils in terms of the plant species, its geographic location, growing and distillation conditions, and the human source of the mental energy that also affects these highly sensitive products of nature. In a way, one could suspect a crystalline action here, in that the essential oils seem not only to transfer energy, but to absorb and hold it, just as a crystal can hold information and give it out. (Think of the first crystal radios, and the computer revolution in Silicon Valley, California — silicon is crystalline.) This phenomenon is well known to scientists who increasingly study crystals with great interest. There's a rumor in some scientific circles that the National Aeronautics and Space Administration (NASA) currently has a program in place where, in "the black room," a huge crystal sits in a pool of purified water, from which information is transferred by the water-memory mechanism. A computer picks up the informational bytes and records them. Scientists watch as information seeps out of the crystal, in much the same way as archaeologists have watched clay tablets with cuneiform writing get dug out of the ground. There is a language, both on the clay tablets and in the crystal.

Deciphering the information is, of course, another matter. Archaeologists have over the years successfully worked on many ancient languages and today scientists are working on an even more ancient code — the language of the universe that is hidden in crystals.

If we think of essential oils as liquid crystals, we should ask ourselves what information has been absorbed by them in terms of energetic transference, including other people's thought forms. Essential oils have many qualities, only some of which we know well and appreciate. It is their chemistry that's best understood, and this is how essential oils are usually defined. At University College in London, Dr. Luca Turin has been working on the vibration rate of aromatic materials, which is a feature of their chemistry. He believes it is the vibration of an aroma molecule that makes it "smell" a certain way, rather than its molecular shape, which was until recently the usual explanation for the smell mechanism (the shape of the aroma molecule "locks" into an olfactory receptor, which sends a message to the brain). Establishing the vibration rate of an aroma molecule involves electron tunneling spectroscopy, which means building up a database of the frequencies of essential oils will take years, according to Dr. Turin.

When working with the aura and chakras, the vibration rate of essential oils may be more important than their chemistry, although they are of course related. Another aspect of their chemistry, or rather their molecular shape, is their ability to refract light — either to the left, or to the right, or not at all.

The electrical frequency of essential oils can be measured in megahertz, although the reading can change dramatically depending on who has handled the oil. At present, it remains an inexact science but one with great potential for working with auras, chakras, and the physical body — when these can also be routinely measured and compared with an optimum scale.

Some people place great emphasis on the color of essential oils for subtle energy therapy. The color of oils can vary quite considerably between different species, from clear to yellow, orange, red, brown, green, and bright blue. Color is one of the most obvious differences between essential oils, and each color has its own vibration, but this is actually a very complex subject and is discussed much further in chapter 10.

Another difference between essential oils is their viscosity, which leads to an area of difference — evaporation rate — that is important when we're working with the human energy fields. The aura is a part of ourselves that is more connected to the spiritual realms than is our physical body. When thinking in energetic terms, we talk about "grounding" a person who might be too "spaced

USING ESSENTIAL OILS IN THE AURIC FIELD	
Method 1	***Method 2***
Put 1 drop of neat essential oil in the center of the palm of one hand, rub the hands together, and smooth around the outside of the body. Start on the side of the body, from the feet, working to the top of the head. Then repeat the movement on the front of the body, feet to head; then on the back, feet to head.	Use the essential oils in the spray/mister method, spraying around the body and over the top of the head. With this method, it is preferable to first combine your essential oils together, making a synergistic blend, and leave them for seven days in a peaceful place, away from electromagnetic activity such as electrical equipment. On the eighth day, using a new perfume mister, put in one ounce of the purest water you can get, which should come in a glass, not plastic, bottle. Add the essential oils and shake well.

ESSENTIAL OILS TO ENERGIZE

Lemon	Eucalyptus
Pine	Basil
Fir	Peppermint
Spruce	Coriander

ENERGIZING AURA-CLEANSING SPRAY

Pine	4 drops
Spruce	5 drops
Fir Needle	5 drops
Basil	3 drops
Lemon	3 drops

ESSENTIAL OILS TO HARMONIZE

Geranium	Ginger
Lavender	Fennel
Petitgrain	Cistus
Mandarin	Juniper
Clary Sage	Orange

HARMONIZING AURA-CLEANSING SPRAY

Geranium	4 drops
Juniper	2 drops
Petitgrain	6 drops
Orange	6 drops
Fennel	1 drop

ESSENTIAL OILS TO AWAKEN THE HIGHER SELF

Frankincense
Neroli
Rose
Jasmine
Linden Blossom

SPIRITUAL CONNECTION AURIC-FIELD SPRAY

Galbanum	1 drop
Frankincense	4 drops
Rose	7 drops
Jasmine	2 drops
Neroli	7 drops

out," almost as if the person could float off into the sky; or about "centering" a person whose energy is dissipated and all over the place; or about "lightening up" a person who is too "heavy" energetically.

There's little point in using a grounding oil on someone who is already grounded to the spot, or lightening up someone who is already so light he or she is practically floating through the ceiling. Many seek to "lighten up," in the sense of realizing spiritual potential. Really, we want to seek balance, and find the spiritual core that is at the heart of that balance.

The evaporation rate of essential oils is an indicator of their quality in terms of energetic frequency. It's not the whole story but a part of it that needs to be considered. In perfumery, the evaporation rate of essential oils is categorized in three ways: top note or quick evaporation; middle note or average rate of evaporation; and base note or slow evaporation, and thus the aroma that most endures. When two or more essential oils are blended together the story becomes more complex. In a particular perfume, for example, an essential oil might be classified as one of the components in the middle note, and in another perfume, it may be a top note. Everything is relative, they say, and when blending essential oils for energetic work that is certainly true.

Each essential oil has its top note, middle note, and base note. You can experience this yourself by putting a drop of any oil on your skin and sniffing it immediately, then five minutes later, half an hour later, and two hours later. Close your eyes and feel how deep each aroma can be.

To compare the evaporation rates of different essential oils you will need a few smelling strips. These can be made out of any absorbent white paper, or even out of natural undyed material. Put a drop of essential oil on three strips, choosing one each from the three evaporation-rate categories, and keep coming back to the strips over a period of time to see how their aromas change. The quicker the evaporation rate, the quicker the aroma molecules have released into the air, and the quicker they can move through and influence the auric field.

EVAPORATION RATES WITHIN THE AURIC FIELD		
Top Note	*Middle Note*	*Base Note*
Aniseed	Bay	Balsam de Peru
Artemisia	Black Pepper	Benzoin
Basil	Cardamom	Cistus
Bergamot	Cedarwood	Galbanum
Cajuput	Chamomile German	Myrrh
Caraway	Chamomile Maroc	Orris Root
Chamomile Roman	Cinnamon Leaf	Patchouli
Citronella	Clary Sage	Sandalwood
Coriander	Clove Bud	Styrax
Eucalyptus Globulus	Cypress	Valerian
Fennel (Sweet)	Geranium	Vetiver
Fir	Ginger	
Frankincense	Helichrysum (Italian Everlasting)	
Juniper	Hyssop	
Lavender	Jasmine	
Lemon	Lemongrass	
Mandarin	Marjoram (Sweet)	
Neroli	Melissa	
Niaouli	Nutmeg	
Orange	Oregano	
Peppermint	Palmarosa	
Petitgrain	Parsley Seed	
Pine	Rose Maroc	
Rose Otto	Rosemary	
Spearmint	Rosewood	
	Sage	
	Tagetes	
	Thyme	
	Turmeric	
	Violet Leaf	
	Yarrow	
	Ylang Ylang	

The colors seen in the auric field are said to reflect the physical, mental, and spiritual aspects of a person. A great deal has been written about this, both in ancient and recent texts, and a summary of what the auric colors are said to indicate follows:

AURIC COLORS	
Color	*Indicates*
Red — *Physicality*	Pain; muscular problems; inflammation; strong emotional states
Orange — *Creativity*	Strong imagination; emotional; feelings; weeping
Yellow — *Rationality*	Strong-willed; frustration; intellectualism; logical; analytical
Green — *Harmony*	Harmony; rested; balanced; reconciliation with past hurts; letting go
Blue — *Peace*	Peace; strength; calm; ease; recognizing true self
Violet/Purple — *Mysticism*	Connecting to higher consciousness; connecting to true self
White — *Spirituality*	Transformation and meeting with the spirit

Part Two

Aromatherapy
and the Spiritual Connection

Chapter 9

Vibrational Aromatherapy

There is nothing less scientific than to deny something because it cannot be explained.

— Dr. Jean Valnet,
in *The Practice of Aromatherapy*

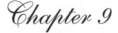AROMATHERAPY *IS* VIBRATIONAL, as it utilizes tools that each have an individual vibration — the aromatic essential oils — that affect living, vibrational people. When I trained in physical therapy and phytotherapy in mainland Europe more years ago than I care to remember, we were taught vibrational theories, as Austrian philosopher Rudolph Steiner had great influence there. Others talked about vibrational aromatherapy in their particular fields, such as biochemist Marguerite Maury, in rejuvenation. Looking back now at the aromatherapy teaching material supplied to students in the early days of aromatherapy, it's clear that vibrations were very much part of the language and concepts taught.

The roots of modern aromatherapy can be found in the intellectual life of Europe in the 1960s, which was very open to the holistic view, not only of the person but of nature and the universe in general. Wholeness was discussed in the broadest of terms. In those days, it was a therapy generally reserved for the wealthy, who could afford the luxury of visits to private European clinics. Physiologist Arnold Taylor brought Maury to England to teach, and under the influence of her style and practice, which included massage and bodywork, aromatherapy developed.

As aromatherapy became more generally known and available, there was the need to validate it by focusing on the physically obvious medicinal qualities of essential oils, and there are hundreds of research papers that can quantify their various properties. Science can now see how aromatherapy works, that there are established physiological mechanisms involved. Moreover, from other more recent work in the area of brain chemistry, science can even explain how aromatherapy can make a person feel good emotionally. These revelations are a long way from how things were thirty years ago, when the term *aromatherapy* was equated with "nice-smells-make-you-feel-good-airy-fairy-psychological-nonsense-and-not-only-that-it's-good-for-the-skin!"

The use of essential oils is now understood to be something more scientifically interesting than perfume. Aromatherapy has gone through this period of acceptance, consolidating the facts established by scientific research with actual practical results, leaving unsaid a whole aspect of our work that could broadly be put under the term *vibrational aromatherapy*. Energetics is what holds it all together.

Those of us who learned aromatherapy when it was seen as a mind-body-spirit, whole-person therapy have always discussed it in terms of vibration and frequency, and some have taught it that way. People who came into the profession when it was going through its very pragmatic "let's be very scientific and talk about the chemical aspect" stage may have bypassed these important aspects. The latest group joining the profession come to it knowing they have to learn the scientific medical facts but not necessarily the vocabulary of energetic aromatherapy — auras, chakras, subtle bodies, energy exchange — as these terms are now more commonly used. There is, however, nothing new about "vibrational," "frequency," or "energetic" aromatherapy. It's been talked about for decades, and known about ever since people mixed fragrant plants and oils together and used them on their bodies, which was tens of centuries ago.

Vibrational aromatherapy is not something that can be practiced alone because it *includes* physical aromatherapy and emotional aromatherapy. They are integral to each other, part of a single whole. To be a holistic aromatherapist you must be an expert in the physical, body and oil; the emotional, body and oil; and the spiritual, body and oil. Holistic aromatherapy is not, therefore, an easy option, although there are those who will set up practice as "energetic" or "vibrational" aromatherapists on the basis that "all illness starts in the etheric." It doesn't matter where the illness starts, the point is that it is there, manifesting in the physical, mental, emotional, or spiritual — or all four. To treat a person energetically, all aspects of a person must be understood. Energetic therapies cannot be shortcuts, bypassing the physical, because vibration *is* part of essential oils and the physical body. The subtle and physical bodies of a person work together like the printer's primary colors — one doesn't make sense of one without the others, and you need all the colors, or bodies, to see the whole. Vibrational or energetic aromatherapy *is* aromatherapy, period.

THE CHAKRAS

In the etheric body there are centers of energy, sometimes described as wheels, or vortices. There are seven main chakras and twenty-one minor ones. Healers often bring one of the minor chakras, the spleen, into the main group of seven, because the spleen is so directly involved in the immune system and in healing the physical body. The main chakras are said to be related to the physical body in the following way:

Crown Center	pineal gland (some say pituitary)
Brow Center	pituitary gland (some say pineal); eyes and brain
Throat Center	speech and hearing; nervous system; thyroid gland; lungs and bronchial tubes; digestive tract
Heart Center	heart and lungs
Solar Plexus	stomach, digestive system
Sacral Center	genital system
Base Center	kidneys, excretory system, adrenal glands

The 21 Minor Chakras

2   by ears, in front, middle
2   above each breast
1   where breast bones meet
2   in palms of the hands
2   in soles of the feet
2   at outer corners of the eyes
2   at gonads
1   close to the liver
1   by the stomach
2   by the spleen
2   at the backs of the knees
1   connected with vagus nerve, near the thymus gland
1   close to the solar plexus

BODY SCANNING

By scanning the body you can determine areas that are misaligned, or lacking in healthy energy flow. The hands are held a couple of inches above the skin and skimmed over the body to feel the general state of the aura and locate areas that are particularly hot or cold, or even clammy. The chakras are most clearly felt as different, and they have above their location an energy that varies from person to person. There is no substitute for actual practice in scanning, by which comparisons can be made of the different feel of auras and chakras. The aura can be felt two inches above the surface of the body, and the chakras at around six to eight inches.

The body has an electromagnetic field that can be registered by mechanical equipment. The therapist can become a living form of that kind of equipment, with practice. One day all therapists may make scanning a preliminary procedure to hands-on therapy, in much the same way neurologists routinely attach electrodes to the surface of heads to help them make a diagnosis, when once such equipment was totally unknown. If we, as therapists, were inert, we couldn't body scan; as it is, we are ourselves electrically sensitive, mechanically able to pick up energy, provided we have been tuned into the practice.

Body scanning simply involves running the palms of both hands over the body of a person, looking for changes in the energy field. This obviously has to be done with great awareness, and I feel it helps to very slightly bounce the hands to feel what resistance is there. If, for example, you feel a hot spot over a shoulder, it could indicate pain or injury, perhaps an old injury that is still manifest in the auric field. Such injuries may not be bothering the person today, but when he or she is fatigued at some time in the future, or undergoing physical, emotional, or spiritual pressure, this old pain may return to the body, even if the injury or wound has "healed" physically. Old wounds can come back to haunt us if, in reality, they never went away — if they got stored in the subtle body under "unfinished business." Working in the subtle body not only identifies such lingering problems, it is the route through which to transform them, by clearing and strengthening the energy field. Chronic physical pain that just will not go away often responds well to anti-inflammatory essential oils, such as chamomile, used in the energetic field preliminary to physically working on the body.

When scanning a body, place the essential oils in your hand, which you move in slow, small circles over the area, hovering just above it. Then, after working on such an area, wash your hands before continuing with the scan. Moving over the body and clearing as much as you possibly can within the subtle body often releases long-buried physical injuries, emotional crises, and trauma. Gradually, layer by layer, impediments holding the client back from complete wellness appear to dissipate, and the person's physical body will be better able to respond to any physical treatment subsequently applied.

All therapists work with the aura and chakras, even if they don't realize it. Every client comes to a therapist with an energy profile. We may talk about it in generally accepted terms, saying, for example, "He has a high energy level," or "He's hyper," or "Her energy level is very low — she needs a boost." These phrases describe a frequency that can now be measured by sophisticated equipment. This energy is subtle, a quality of the energy field that is unseen by the naked eye, but tangible nonetheless. We might find ourselves saying of a person operating from one chakra area more than the others, "His emotional pain is deep in the belly," or "Her heart is broken," or "His head rules his heart." All these are imbalances. Ideally, a person needs all their chakras, all their body areas and energies, working in a vibrant clear way, unfettered by emotional and physical pain. Through no fault of their own, only circumstance, people may have become imbalanced in terms of energy. Perhaps their parents were emotionally cold, which disallowed the flowering of a warm and vibrant heart — a less active heart chakra. People can become imbalanced for countless reasons; a therapist's job is to provide the environment in which energy balance and healing can take place.

To begin with, simply look for the general energy level, and work to balance that. With experience, you'll come to know the energy of the various chakras and be able to see which have an excess energy or a depletion in these various areas. You can look for heat, cold, lack of energy, excess of energy, and something very tangible, the *feel* of the aura, which can in cases of impoverished mental and emotional habits, or ill health, be felt as a clammy, gooey cloud.

Chakras relate to particular vertebrae, which in turn relate to particular nerves and organs. By feeling the chakra energy, you can often cross-reference, and question the client about the health of relevant areas of the body. People do not mean to hold information back; they might not think it very important, having more pressing problems on their mind, or they might simply have forgotten about a past health event, or seemingly unrelated one. By scanning the aura above the surface of the body, you have another diagnostic tool at your disposal, which, with good communication with a person, can often reveal problems hidden deep within the body.

The chakras listed in the far left column of the following chart pertain to the designated body areas and their related disorders on the right. Where there is deficiency or excess in the energy/function of one chakra, it will be compensated for by the opposite action in the adjacent chakras. The spleen chakra, usually considered a minor chakra, has been included here because it actually has a major action on the physical energetic body. It often overlinks with the solar plexus chakra, there being a close energy-compensation action between the two, which is why when the solar plexus is depressed by impoverished emotions, the spleen is given more work to do. In order for the upper chakras to resonate with clarity, the lower chakras need balancing first, providing a strong scaffolding for the clear reception and transmission to and from the upper chakras. The radiation of energy from any particular chakra blends with the energy of those adjacent to it, to a greater or lesser degree depending on the proximity of the adjacent chakra.

CHAKRAS AND RELATED BODY AREAS				
Chakra	*Location*	*Vertebra(e)*	*Nerves Affected*	*Physical Disorders*
Crown Chakra	Situated at fontanelle; affects to 1C	1C	Blood supply to the head; scalp; bones of the face; brain; pituitary gland; inner and middle ear; sympathetic nervous system	Headaches; anxiety; insomnia; nervous breakdown; amnesia; chronic tiredness; dizziness/vertigo; high blood pressure; migraine
Brow Chakra	Situated at atlas; affects 2C to 4C	2C	Eyes and optic nerves; sinuses; mastoid bones; auditory nerve; forehead; tongue	Sinus problems; deafness; allergies; eye conditions; earaches; feeling faint
		3C	Face bones; cheeks; teeth; trifacial nerve; outer ear	Neuralgia; neuritis; eczema; skin complaints
		4C	Lips; mouth; nose; eustachian tubes	Sinus problems; adenoids; hay fever; anosmia; lip ulceration; nose polyps
Throat Chakra	Situated at 5C; affects 3C to 7C	5C	Neck glands; vocal cords; pharynx	Laryngitis; throat conditions; swollen glands; frequent loss of voice; inability to swallow; goiter
		6C	Tonsils; neck muscles; shoulders	Neck pains; upper arm pains; frequent coughing; tickles in throat; stiffness in shoulders
		7C	Thyroid gland; bursae in the shoulders; the elbows	Bursitis; hyperthyroidism; hypothyroidism; hormonal problems

CHARKAS AND RELATED BODY AREAS (CONT.)				
Chakra	*Location*	*Vertebra(e)*	*Nerves Affected*	*Physical Disorders*
Throat Chakra (cont.)	Situated at 5C; affects 3C to 7C	1T	Esophagus and trachea; fingers; hands; wrists; arms up to the elbow	Asthma; breathing difficulties; shortness of breath; frequent coughing; aches or pains in lower arms and hands; backache
Heart Chakra	Situated at 2T; affects 7C to 4T	2T	Heart; heart valves; coronary arteries; thymus gland	Heart conditions; chest pains; angina; circulation problems; high cholesterol; palpitations
		3T	Lungs; bronchial tubes; pleura; chest; breast	Respiratory problems; lung congestion; breathing difficulties; chest and breast pain; mastitis; breast cysts
		4T	Gall bladder; common duct	Gall bladder disorders, including stones; persistent viral infections; digestive problems; inability to absorb nutrients
Solar Plexus Chakra	Situated at 5T; affects 3T to 8T	5T	Blood; liver; solar plexus	Liver conditions; low blood pressure; anemia; circulatory conditions; autoimmune disease; rheumatism; persistent viral infections; blood disorders; emotional crises
		6T	Stomach	Digestive problems; frequent indigestion; heartburn; dyspepsia; lack of appetite; hiatal hernia; nausea
		7T	Pancreas; islets of Langerhans; duodenum	Ulceration; gastric conditions; diabetes; digestive problems; hormonal disorders; certain viral infections
Spleen Chakra	Situated at 8T; affects 8T to 12T	8T	Spleen; diaphragm	Lowered immunity; blood disorders; anemia; emotional crises

CHAKRAS AND RELATED BODY AREAS (CONT.)				
Chakra	*Location*	*Vertebra(e)*	*Nerves Affected*	*Physical Disorders*
Spleen Chakra (cont.)	Situated at 8T; affects 8T to 12T	9T	Adrenal glands	Hormonal conditions; inflammatory conditions; immune system problems; stress; tension
		10T	Kidneys	Kidney problems, including stones; chronic tiredness; nephritis; diabetes; drowsiness; nausea
		11T	Kidneys; ureters	Urinary problems; cystitis; prostate problems; hypertension; cysts
		12T	Lymphatic-circulation; small intestines; fallopian tubes	Crohn's disease; parasitic infection; irritable bowel syndrome; abdominal cramps; vomiting; nausea; lowered immunity; circulatory problems; infertility (female); salpingitis
		1L	Large intestines (colon); inguinal rings	Diverticular disease; colitis; constipation; excessive gas; diarrhea; intestinal cramping; varicose veins
		2L	Abdomen; appendix; upper leg; cecum	Abdominal cramps; breathing difficulties; excessive acid; varicose veins
		3L	Uterus; ovaries or testicles; sex organs; bladder; knee	Menstrual problems; endometriosis; menopausal problems; infertility; joint problems; impotence (male); hemorrhoids
		4L	Muscles of the lower back; sciatic nerve; prostate gland	Prostate problems, including difficulty in urinating (male); back pain; sciatic pain; lumbago; leg aches and pains

CHAKRAS AND RELATED BODY AREAS (CONT.)				
Chakra	*Location*	*Vertebra(e)*	*Nerves Affected*	*Physical Disorders*
Sacral Chakra	Situated at 5L; affects 12T to sacrum	5L	Lower legs; ankles; feet; toes	Poor circulation in lower torso and legs; edema in legs; weakness in legs; leg cramps; sciatic pain
		Sacrum	Buttocks; hip bones	Sciatic pain; sacroiliac misalignments; spinal curvature; skeletal conditions
Base Chakra	Situated at coccyx; affects 9T to coccyx	Coccyx	Rectum; anus	Anal itching (puritus); hemorrhoids; anal fissures; constipation; uterine prolapse; prostate problems

ESSENTIAL OILS FOR THE CHAKRAS

Crown Chakra

Neroli, Rose, Frankincense

Brow Chakra

Rosemary, Juniper, Hyacinth, Lemon, Pine, Angelica Seed

Throat Chakra

Chamomile, Linden Blossom, Cypress, Petitgrain, Basil, Peppermint, Hyssop, Rosewood, Rosemary

Heart Chakra

Rose Maroc, Bergamot, Melissa, Ylang Ylang, Mandarin, Tangerine, Geranium, Jasmine, Lavender

Solar Plexus & Spleen Chakras

Juniper, Cedarwood, Coriander, Black Pepper, Lime, Hyssop, Marjoram, Cardamom

Sacral Chakra

Sandalwood, Clary Sage, Fennel, Cardamom, Elemi, Benzoin

Base Chakra

Myrrh, Patchouli, Vetiver, Rosewood, Thyme, Balsam de Peru

USING VIBRATIONAL AROMATHERAPY IN TREATMENT

Whether the treatment is professional or nonprofessional, it takes thought and planning. For those professionals who are contemplating incorporating energetic, or vibrational, aromatherapy into their practice, setting the right environment helps create an atmosphere of a spiritual haven, even in your usual practice room.

Music

Some therapists choose to have music playing during treatments, and others do not. It really depends on how the therapist feels, rather than the client, unless, of course, the client dislikes the chosen musical selection. It's surprising how opinions vary on which music is relaxing and which is not, so choose carefully.

Sounds

Some therapists like to include sound, such as singing or crystal bowls, gongs, or tapes that claim to synchronize, or attune, the human aura. Sounds "clear" a room, changing its energy very quickly. This is most often done at the beginning or end of an individual treatment, or the working day. For those who work as clinical aromatherapists, using anything other than their usual medical skills not only takes up valuable time, but also might seem just a little too New Age. I was told by a sound expert that sound memories, as vibration or sound waves, can become embedded in the fabric of buildings, which made me think about sound and music in a different way. Now, to clear away the conversations of the day, the "informational clutter," I might ring a bell, clang a gong, or even simply strike a glass. Apparently that does the trick.

Color

Color — including white — is applied on a practitioner's walls, but it is equally present in towels, the couch, or massage-table coverings, and in pictures and plants. Try to create a haven of peace and tranquillity that feels fresh and enlivening at the same time. Pictures and accessories can provide a splash of color while the rest of the furnishings can be chosen to produce a peaceful feel. There are many helpful books on this subject.

Aromas

Constantly using different aromas in a room presents a real conundrum for many therapists. A person may have been treated for a rheumatic condition with oils that are a completely different requirement, and aroma, than those needed for the next patient who has, say, an anxiety crisis regarding the inability to feel any type of spirituality — a common occurrence these days.

What can you do, especially as many rooms do not have a window that can be opened? Extractor fans used for five to ten minutes between treatments seem to be the most effective solution. Those who use air conditioners may find the atmosphere is effectively dealt with through this system. An ionizer is another way in which an atmosphere can be changed. Background radiation is another consideration, and there are now several companies that sell machines that are said to stabilize the frequencies, deflect them, or neutralize the "field incoherence."

Accessories

According to feng shui, large crystals placed in the corners of the room, and mirrors that face doors, deflect energy. Lots of green, living plants and running water also help. Flowers and floating candles in a bowl would pretty up any area. The lighting should be arranged so that it does not shine directly on the client.

Treatment

The room is ready, the energies are right, the sound waves have been cleared, and all is in harmony and peace. The consultation is complete, the planned treatment is compatible with the medical history and psychological profile, and an aromatherapy treatment with the additional vibrational work is to take place.

To begin with, the client should be lying on his or her front so that work can begin on the back. Body scanning is done, and if an area of either hot or cold is located, the therapist can harmonize the energy by moving the palms of both hands in very slow circular movements over the area. Then the hands are gently lowered through the energetic field onto the body, and that position is held for a while. This area can then be worked on directly using the essential oil blend already prepared for the client, before continuing with the body scan, if that is not yet finished, or continuing with normal treatment practice.

At what you judge to be the appropriate time, you can balance the chakras, starting very gently at the solar plexus where the emotions are centered. Beyond this, if using the chakras in a treatment, much depends on the particular client and condition. Although many people suggest working up the chakra system, or down, I personally first work downward from the solar plexus to the sacrum, until balance is achieved, then from the top crown chakra I work downward toward the solar plexus, where any emotional problems can again be soothed and calmed. Finally, I check that all chakras, from base to crown, are in balance.

Many people are neglectful of one half of their body or the other, depending on their personality, life situation, and health, and this system helps in the awakening and acknowledgment process. During the scanning and balancing procedure, physical problems such as muscular armory, pain, or misalignment can be corrected as much as possible using the usual physical treatment methods.

When the client is turned over on his or her back, treatment continues with scanning once again, and any ailments or energy still not in balance can be harmonized. The treatment should finish with the head being gently cradled in the hands.

As a therapist you should take into account the position of the chakras in relation to the vertebrae and their associated organs, and in relation to the sympathetic and parasympathetic nervous systems. Please refer to the previous chart. Another factor in treatment is the emotional muscular sites, the places where particular emotions are held in the musculature, as shown in the diagrams on the following pages. The emotions held in the muscles may in fact alter the energetic field and could give a false reading if not taken into account.

Essential oils appropriate to the mind, body, spirit, and character of the person should be chosen with care, taking into account the psycho-spiritual aspects and interactions of the individual oils.

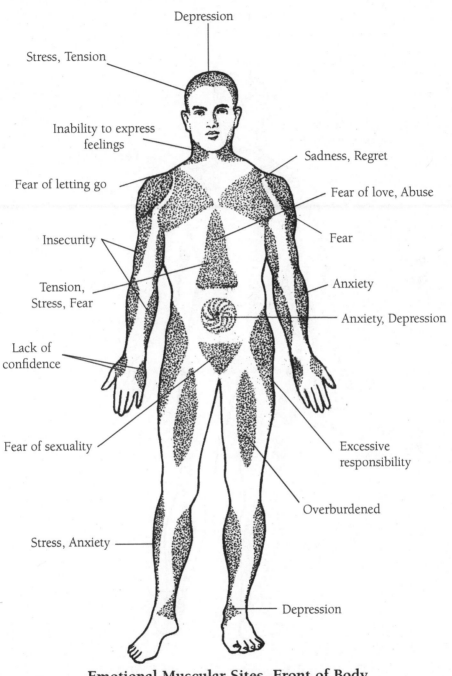

Depression

Stress, Tension

Inability to express
feelings

Sadness, Regret

Fear of letting go

Fear of love, Abuse

Fear

Insecurity

Tension,
Stress, Fear

Anxiety

Anxiety, Depression

Lack of
confidence

Fear of sexuality

Excessive
responsibility

Overburdened

Stress, Anxiety

Depression

Emotional Muscular Sites, Front of Body
(Illustration from *The Fragrant Mind* by Valerie Ann Worwood, New World Library, 1996)

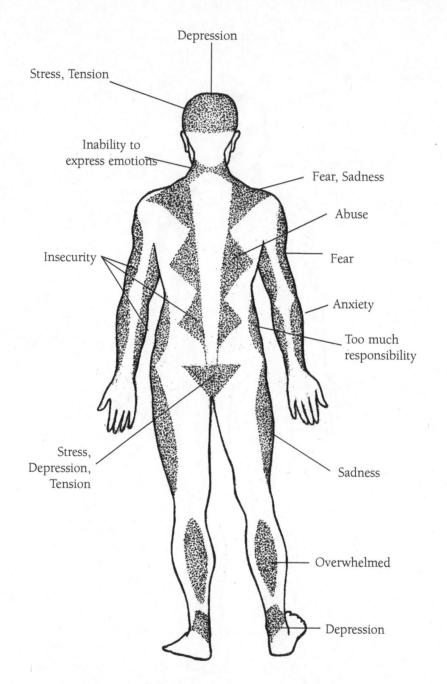

Emotional Muscular Sites, Back of Body

(Illustration from *The Fragrant Mind* by Valerie Ann Worwood, New World Library, 1996)

Miasms

The man who invented modern homeopathy, Samuel Hahnemann (1755–1843) was the first to identify miasms, which are basic vibrational patterns of disease. Miasms are said to have their origin in the subtle, or auric, field, and set up patterns in an individual's body, mind, and personality, causing preset physical or emotional reactions or behavior. The manifestation of miasms are through the subatomic, atomic, molecular, electromagnetic, biochemical, physiological, and psychological energetic pathways. Some people believe miasms can be inherited genetically, or even transferred from one person to another by resonance, that is by being close to a person who has one. A miasm can also be acquired from our parents or in the womb, through the intelligence of the genetic code, in cellular memory, or through emotional trauma or pollution. Miasms tend to show themselves when a person is very tired or under stress. They could be detected in the energetic field and be mistaken for an energetic manifestation of a physical disorder. For example, you might detect bad energy flow in the lower half of the left leg and ask, "Do you have circulation problems here?" The client responds, "No, never." On further questioning, however, you may find that the grandfather had gangrene in the left leg, which was amputated at the knee, and that the father got mysterious pains in the same area whenever he got tired. This is what is meant by miasms — the carrying forward of physical and emotional pain, albeit in reduced form.

Energies

There is no doubt that essential oils affect the aura and chakras. However, they have a different influence, depending on the person receiving them and the person administering them, in terms of how their vibratory rates interact with the fragrance. For example, if the fragrance is of a higher frequency than the person using or administering the oil at that particular time, then the interaction is going to be slower and at a different rate than it would be with persons who are clear-minded and full of energy. The vibrational level of a person could be reduced by stress, ill health, or even a particular mind frame.

The essential oils do not themselves directly harmonize the auric, or energetic, field. The aromatic molecule's energy interacts with the energetic and subtle anatomy of the person, their fragrance molecules stirring, agitating, electrically boosting, or in some other way stimulating the human energetic fields, allowing them to reorganize and harmonize *themselves*.

It could be that diffused oils also react in this way, weaving a way through the energetic field, affecting the physical through the olfactory nerves. Perhaps we smell with our energetic fields and, because of that, science finds it so difficult to gather the information needed to decipher and decode how the sense of smell actually works, and how it has such a profound effect on our minds and spiritual sense of being.

Any treatment using energetics aims to align all bodily currents — physically, emotionally, and spiritually. The physical affects the emotional and the psycho-spiritual connections, and the reverse is also true.

Healing the Spiritual Crisis

Today many people suffer because of the psycho-spiritual aspects of life. Just getting from one day to the next is a major battle for many people. And as time goes on life gets harder, faster, and more stressful. Life is no longer simple, and as we try to do the right thing by our family, friends, workmates, and ourselves, we often find ourselves facing opposition from all manner of officialdom. How do we cope when half the world seems to be driven by unspiritual factors?

All this often results in a psycho-spiritual crisis, raising questions such as "What is the meaning of it all?" and "How can I go on?" Some people might argue that their religion/movement/sect/belief has the answer, point to their religious book, and say, "That is the way." But in this day of global communication, there are many books and many ways to choose from. Perhaps it is wise to bear in mind the old saying "There are many routes to the same place."

Sometimes I watch the TV programs about the arms industry, global warming, or starvation (when there is enough food to go around), and people dying through lack of medicine (when we could make more), and I wonder if I am on the same planet as all this. We can say "We are all equal," but in this real world, in many respects we are not. Is it any wonder that we've all — every one of us — picked up on the vibrations and frequency of psycho-spiritual suffering? I see many people who feel a deep sense of helplessness and powerlessness, regardless of their spiritual beliefs.

So how are we to deal with it? There are some basic, preliminary steps, each one huge and a great personal challenge:

1. Develop the core of love in our hearts so that it fills our being.
2. Forgive, for not to do so only hurts ourselves.
3. Release anger, as that only sets up the body for disease.
4. Remove ourselves from any source of abuse, which depresses the spirit.

No spiritual crisis can be healed by another person. We can be guided, certainly, but ultimately only we can heal our own spiritual crises by taking time to sit and really enter into our inner beings, our inner selves. For me, essential oils have always been, in their own way, a reference point for focus. They allow me time and space for the inner search, and I use a special blend unique to myself, to contemplate, forgive, and make the spiritual connection.

Fragrances help concentrate the mind and change it from a confused cacophony of negativity into a stilled surety of harmony and peace. There within us is this quietude, and it can expand. We can even get beyond our own everyday concerns and perspectives, and see another's point of view. Moreover, fragrances are healing. The natural, God-given, fragrant plant material helps heal the psycho-spiritual connection and can allow us, if only for a brief moment or two, to be free enough to reach out mentally to our higher selves, guiding us beyond this plane of existence to understanding and love.

One very practical aspect of this process is that fragrance can be carried with us anywhere. I've sniffed my special spiritual aroma from a handkerchief on rush-hour underground trains and on airplane flights. Wherever I am, and whatever is going on, I can immediately enter that place of superawareness, far more quickly than by any other route.

Finding a fragrance or making a blend you particularly enjoy is not hard. There are many essential oils to choose from, and finding a fragrance that has a special spiritual effect may take a little time, but it's worth it.

Some people are afraid of the aromas, almost as if they fear connecting into their true selves, because aromas can be very illuminating and revealing. Possibly the reason for this is that they don't like the aromas available to them, but if the "right" (right for them) aroma can be found, they'll love it — deeply. These are best described as potential psycho-spiritual barriers, once expressed to me in the following way: "Intuitively I knew the aromas would bring me to a place within myself, where body and spirit meet, and I was frightened to reach that place because I was ashamed that I'd been so horrible in my life, and was terrified of what I would feel if the defenses were let down. I could imagine it would be wonderful, but what if it wasn't?" This person, Allan, decided after a while that he did love the smells after all, and having had a wonderful experience with them, chose a focusing spiritual oil blend for himself, to give comfort and to help him make contact with the higher self.

Choose your oils from the essential oil profiles, blend carefully, or to start off with enlist the help of someone who has blending experience. Once discovered, keep the formula to yourself, because each blend, like each individual, will be unique — a personal refuge and connection to the fragrant heavens.

THE SEVEN MAIN CHAKRAS

1ST CHAKRA
Modern Name (Root or) Base chakra
Sanskrit Name Muladhara or Guda chakra
Situated Back of the rectum, coccyx
Color Red
Petals Four energy vortices
Element Earth or solids
This chakra needs to be cleansed and purified both emotionally and physically before any of the others; it is the first to be activated. The support chakra.
Physical Associations Kidneys; excretion; spine
Associated Glands Adrenal glands
Associated Emotions Fear; obsessive/compulsive behavior; protective instincts
Weakness Nonattachment; nervous instability

2ND CHAKRA
Modern Name Sacral chakra
Sanskrit Name Indra or Swada or Svadasthan chakra
Situated Near the sacral bone (above first lumbar)
Color Orange (some older texts say yellow)
Petals Six energy vortices
Element Water
It controls the creation of the physical form. Sexual energy and all its desires.
Physical Associations • Sexual reproduction • Balance between estrogen, progesterone, testosterone • Liquids within the body: blood, urine, lymph, mucus, semen
Associated Glands Gonads: ovaries, testicles
Associated Emotions Desire; jealousy
Weakness Lust; addictions; anger; pride; aggression

3RD CHAKRA

Modern Name
Solar Plexus chakra

Sanskrit Name
Manipurak or Nabi chakra

Situated
Near the solar plexus at the umbilicus (7th and 8th thoracic vertebrae)

Color
Yellow

Petals
Eight energy vortices

Element
Fire

Suggestive of the sun, which is also needed for the metabolism of plant and human life.

Physical Associations
- Stomach; digestive system; spleen
- Metabolism: keeps the balance between anabolic-catabolic (the building up of simple material into complex substances; and the breaking down of complex substances into simple ones)
- Heat-regulation control
- Endocrine digestive processes; sugar metabolism; production of insulin

Associated Gland
Pancreas

Associated Emotions
Warmth; nurturing; fiery nature

Weakness
Emotional instability; skin eruptions

4TH CHAKRA

Modern Name
Heart chakra

Sanskrit Name
Anahata chakra

Situated
Between the breasts (5th thoracic)

Color
Green

Petals
Twelve energy vortices

Element
Earth/Air

The protector and distributor of energy for the lower chakras.

Physical Associations
- Heart; blood circulation
- Lung; respiration
- The immune system; thymosin hormones
- Touch/sensation

Associated Gland
Thymus

Associated Emotions
Love; compassion; protectiveness

Weakness
Heart problems; overprotectiveness; attachment; greed; anger; hyperimmune reactions, including rheumatoid arthritis

THE SEVEN MAIN CHAKRAS (CONT.)

5TH CHAKRA

Modern Name
Throat chakra

Sanskrit Name
Kanth or Vishudhi chakra

Situated
Near the cervical plexus
(3rd cervical vertebra)

Color Blue

Petals
Sixteen energy vortices

Element
Fire/Water/Air (ether)

- *It has an energy field known as akash, which keeps the lower energy currents running smoothly and energizes rational thought.*
- *Where intelligence focuses in creativity, especially of the spoken/written word.*
- *Genital/reproductive system can be worked on from this center.*

Physical Associations
- Vocal cords
- Pulmonary and bronchial systems
- Nervous system

Associated Glands
Thyroid and parathyroid

Associated Emotions
Honesty or dishonesty; criticism

Weakness
Imbalances of all kinds: vertigo, allergies, anemia; menstrual problems; sore throat, laryngitis

6TH CHAKRA

Modern Name
Brow chakra

Sanskrit Name
Ajuna or Do Dal Kanwal chakra

Situated
Between the eyes in the middle of the forehead

Color Purple or violet

Petals
Two energy vortices

Element
Air (ether)

- *"The third eye," where mind and spirit meet within the physical context. The energy from this point spreads into every cell of the body.*
- *All other chakras are dependent upon, and ruled by, this.*
- *Cognition: consciousness and subconsciousness.*
- *This area links the subtle energy field for the whole body.*

Physical Associations
- Sense of smell
- Brain, eyes, nose, ears

Associated Glands
Pituitary; pineal

Associated Emotions
Imagination; idealism; love

Weakness
Pessimism; self-pity; migraine; sleeplessness; catarrh; sinus problems; hay fever

7TH CHAKRA

Modern Name

Crown chakra

Sanskrit Name

Sahasrara chakra

Situated

Top of the head
(approached via base of skull)

Color

White or white-gold

Petals

Twelve energy vortices

Element

None: Some say magnesium,
speech, or spirit

*All energies running through subtle
meridians in our bodies — such as chi
and prana — stop here. It is thought
meridians and the acupuncture points,
or nadirs, were discovered through
opening of the crown chakra and higher
consciousness.*

Physical Associations

Malfunctions of pituitary gland

Associated Glands

Pineal; pituitary

Associated Emotion

Emotional imbalance

Weakness

Coma; epilepsy

THE FRAGRANT SYMPHONY

Sound and fragrance are expressions of vibration, as is color. All three have a similarity in that these vibrations can be put together, creating something that is more than the sum of the parts. Musical notes can be put together to create chords and melody, and several pigments can be put together to create new colors and beautiful pictures. Fragrance is similar: several aromas can be blended to create the fragrant symphony.

Blending is an art, accomplished in the world of fragrance by G. W. Septimus Piesse, author of *The Art of Perfumery*, published in 1856. He introduced the idea of thinking of fragrance in terms of musical notes and created the "Gamut of Odors," a comparative scale:

THE GAMUT OF ODORS

TREBLE (or G Clef)		BASE (or F Clef)	
F	Civet	C	Rose
E	Verbena	B	Cinnamon
D	Citronella	A	Tolu
C	Pineapple	G	Sweet Pea
B	Peppermint	F	Musk
A	Lavender	E	Orris
G	Magnolia	D	Heliotrope
F	Ambergris	C	Geranium
E	Cedrat (Lemon)	B	Stocks and Pinks (Carnation)
D	Bergamot	A	Balsam de Peru
C	Jasmine	G	Pergalaria
B	Mint	F	Castor
A	Tonka Bean	E	Calamus
G	Syringa (Mock Orange Flower)	D	Clematis
F	Jonquil	C	Santal (Sandalwood)
E	Portugal (Orange)	B	Clove
D	Almond	A	Storax
C	Camphor	G	Frangipani (*Plumeria alba*)
B	Southernwood	F	Benzoin
A	Vernal Grass (New Hay)	E	Wallflower
G	Orange Flower	D	Vanilla
F	Tuberose	C	Patchouli
E	Acacia		
D	Violet		

Piesse wrote:

> Scents, like sounds, appear to influence the olfactory nerve in certain degrees. There is, as it were, an octave of odors like an octave in music; certain odors coincide, like the keys of an instrument. Such as almond, heliotrope, vanilla, and orange blossom blend together, each producing different degrees of a nearly similar impression. Again, we have citron, lemon, orange peel, and verbena, forming a higher octave of smells, which blend in a similar manner. The metaphor is completed by what we are pleased to call semi-odors, such as rose and rose-geranium for the half note; petitgrain, neroli, a black key, followed by fleur d'orange. . . .

Piesse quoted a magazine article that made the following points: Music follows a mathematical law depending on nature, who does not waste power and becomes more simple the better she is understood. The final hypothesis was that "the whole of the pleasures of the sense of smell will be found to depend upon cognate laws."

In the future, as the science of vibrational aroma expands, we may discover new aromatic laws that can guide us when blending two or more fragrances, in proportions that follow these underlying principles, to create a perfect harmony. In the meantime, we rely upon our deep knowledge and appreciation of individual aromas. We tune in to their vibration and tone knowing what can be joined together without there being a discordant note, or a smothering of one by another.

Think of an insensitive drummer sitting behind a band crashing away noisily, drowning out the other instruments. Essential oils can do the same thing — drown out the sounds of others in a blend. We did not invent or create essential oils, but when blending them, we are the composer, the conductor, and the sound engineer. It is up to us to know the capacity and beauty of each instrument in our orchestra, and to know when it is time to bring each beautiful tool of the heavens into our symphony.

Chapter 10

Energetic Aromatherapy

Students make up their oils according to the same formulation, using the same essential oils, vegetable oils, and bottles under the same atmospheric conditions. Yet when the finished products are compared, each one is slightly different. It is impossible for two people to reproduce exactly the same thing because each person has different hands and a different electromagnetic field, both of which influence the finished product.
— Micheline Arcier, *Aromatherapy*

ESSENTIAL OILS BOTH GIVE AND RECEIVE ENERGY, as seen in the PIP aura pictures of essential oils taken by Harry Oldfield, and as we know from our own experience. Essential oils can be energetically measured by more conventional means, in megahertz. Each megahertz equals one million oscillations per second, being the frequency of their vibrational motion. However, the megahertz number arrived at by using specialist equipment does not really tell us very much because the frequency of any one essential oil is changed dramatically when it comes into contact with other energies — people, for example.

I took some essential oils to Bruce Tanio, an agricultural scientist and inventor, who has the apparatus to test the frequencies of essential oils. The reading from a rose bulgar was 28 megahertz, but after I'd held the bottle for a while, it's reading was 202 megahertz. That's quite a difference! Another bottle of rose bulgar, from another source and held in another hand, might produce two readings dissimilar to my own. As Tanio remarked, "There is no consistency in the frequency of essential oils."

The vocabulary of energy work is expanding. Tanio talks of a "symphony of frequencies occurring in the cells" and a "resonant harmonic factor," for example. As seen in other scientists' works, the energy field of a person extends outside the confines of the physical form. That field, and the body it encloses, can be changed by the introduction of other energy forces.

There has been a great deal of publicity about the negative influences of magnetic waves in the form of energy on human cells and psyche by, for example, cellular phones, microwaves, and power cables. Another electrical influence that affects humans are the ions in the atmosphere — to put it simply, negative ions make us feel good, and positive ions make us feel not so good. Positive ions — the not-so-good ones (just to be confusing) — can be created seasonally in certain geographic locations, when a strong wind comes into contact with a mountain range with a particular shape configuration. This happens for a month each year in Geneva, Switzerland, and with the Santa Ana winds in Southern California, for example. They make people feel irritable, even aggressive, and sometimes unwell — particularly with headaches, migraines, allergies, and digestive and respiratory problems. Working at the University of California in Los Angeles, Dr. Valerie Hunt recorded the fact that when the Santa Anas were blowing, the human energy field became small. She writes, "It is as though the negative auric field splits away from the body, attracted by the high positive charge of the atmosphere."

On the other hand, a high incidence of negative ions makes us feel good, vitalized, giving us a positive frame of mind. We can inhale negative ions while taking a shower, or when near a waterfall or the sea, or in the mountains, and discharge positive ions into the ground when walking barefoot on the grass. We can even purchase negative ions, or at least the "ionizers" that create them. Dr. Valerie Hunt found that the energy field of subjects expanded when measured near the sea or on a mountain and suggests this is due to the increased negative ions in the atmosphere at these locations.

Another way to positively affect the human energy field is to use essential oils, those vibrational marvels of nature. Many healers have been discovering this, and incorporate them in their practice. This is what this chapter is about: using essential oils for healing. The principles of working with energetic aromatherapy outlined here will apply to any healing modality.

If you are not trained in aromatherapy, don't use essential oils directly on the body of another person. When working with energy, there is absolutely no need. There are many other methods of using essential oils that are very effective for energy work, described throughout the various sections of this book.

All aromas have the potential to evoke memories in a person, depending on what has happened to him or her in the past. The healer has no way of knowing which aromas may invoke a memory, and the client may not even know until they smell it. Those memories may not always be happy ones, and may be associated with someone the client knows and has a hard time with, or even with someone who has passed on and for whom they are still grieving. Memories, either the client's or the healer's, may alter the energetic response. The aromatic environment needs, then, to be either bland or guided by a sensitive, conscious mind.

The haphazard or thoughtless introduction of aroma into the healing room can occur through the products we use on a daily basis, such as perfumed soaps, hand creams, deodorants, cologne, hair products, and through powdered laundry soap and fabric conditioners — in linens or towels, for example. In some healing modalities, two or three people may be involved in the energetic work, and in these cases, aromatic overload could become a problem. In addition, people may have an aversion to certain unnatural product ingredients and aromas. There are now many natural unfragranced personal care products on the market, including glycerin soaps, and these could be used when healing.

Some people go to healers not because anything is wrong with them but as a preventive "workout." Most, however, see healers for a specific reason or two. When choosing essential oils for a particular person, these reasons — along with his or her physical, emotional, mental, and spiritual needs — must be taken into consideration. Energy work aims for flow and interaction, and anything that facilitates this is welcome. Refer to chapter 11, where the therapeutic, emotional, and spiritual qualities of essential oils can be found in their individual profiles. There are many oils to choose from. Before commencing, put a drop or just a smear of your chosen essential oil on the end of a smelling strip and ask the client if he or she likes it, or at least does not have an aversion to it.

Essential oils can also be used in another way: on the healer to increase his or her ability to work energetically. Points and practical suggestions are made to this effect later in this chapter. Clearly though, if there is more than one healer, they will have to be consulted on the choice of essential oils used in room diffusers.

The refreshing tree essential oils of pine, spruce, fir, and cypress are usually received well in a waiting area, especially if electrical equipment is nearby, such as computers, clocks, radios, photocopiers, microwaves, and the ubiquitous mobile phone. When using essential oils in a diffuser in the waiting room, consider the clients you are seeing that day, refer to the profiles, and then make a sensitive choice. Use only small amounts to create a light and gentle fragrant background.

ESSENTIAL OILS AND SPIRITUAL HEALING

Spiritual healers who "lay hands" on patients may or may not actually touch the body. Most work in the auric field with their hands a few inches from the surface. However, healers always say that the healing energies come from outside themselves, and that they are merely a channel for them. Most usually, the source of this healing energy is said to be "God," "the divine power," "universal energy," or "the cosmic intelligence." Essential oils can be incorporated into any form of subtle healing technique, by working within the subtle bodies of a person. As with all energetic aromatherapy, there is no need to apply essential oils directly on the skin.

When approaching any client, have nonjudgmental loving intention and clarity of thought, a clear idea of what you are setting out to achieve, and a concrete course of action. From the client records you should know what physical, emotional, and spiritual needs the client has, and will have your repertoire of hand positions and other particular healing practices. Using essential oils adds another layer to this energetic work, and on that level you need to know how you are going to achieve your aim, by learning about the oils in terms of their physical, emotional, and spiritual properties. The profiles in the next chapter will help you with this information. To "intuit" an essential oil, one first needs a wealth of information maintained in the psyche from which that inspirational knowledge can evolve.

Healers will be acutely aware that physical dysfunctions can be caused by intense anxiety and stress, for example, and there are enough essential oils to choose from that one can be found to help with the emotional cause and physical symptom concurrently, allowing the spiritual to shine through. Not all illness is mind or emotion based. People get ill for all sorts of reasons that have little or nothing to do with them, such as toxic contamination at work, which might be chemical or electromagnetic, and encountered recently or long ago; and accidental injury, which might be recent, or hardly remembered as it occurred so far in the past.

There are three main ways to use essential oils in spiritual healing, with each involving different methods:

- In the room (healing room or waiting room)
- In the auric field of the client
- On yourself, the healer

In the Room

If you feel that using essential oils in the treatment room will interrupt your concentration, consider using them in the waiting room. The aromas will relax and open the hearts of people, making them more receptive to healing.

The usual type of diffuser or burner has a candle, which should be extinguished if the room is left unattended. Also available are electrical ceramic and fan models. Two or three drops is usually sufficient to provide the subtle fragrant background. Unless you want the energy to be very grounded, don't use myrrh or the other base vibrational or heavy oils in a waiting room.

It's generally unnecessary to use blends while giving any type of spiritual healing, which has its own dynamic flow. The essential oils are used to facilitate and complement that flow, by creating a space in which healing can take place, and singular oils have a simplicity and clarity that is appropriate to this process. The choice of singular oil can, of course, change over time.

In the Auric Field of the Client

Making an appropriate essential oil choice for the client from his or her general demeanor involves, as far as the individual healer's abilities allow, constructing a mental light-image of physical, emotional, and spiritual aspects of the client's well-being, his or her subtle bodies, chakras, and aura. When this broader overview has emerged, and an increasingly broad knowledge of essential oils gained, more appropriate choices of essential oil can be made.

Choose one of the following methods before beginning the healing process:

- Put one drop of essential oil on a small piece of white paper or cloth. Place it in the center of the palm of your hand, then cover it with the other hand. Rub your hands together lightly, then discard the paper.
- Wash your hands as usual before commencing treatment. Then fill a sink or bowl halfway with water, add a drop or two of essential oil, and swish it around. Rinse your hands in this water and lightly pat them dry.
- Have a preprepared floral water, as described in the Methods of Use section in chapter 2. Spray your hands with it.
- Essential oils can be put on the floor under the treatment couch, in line with one or more chakras. They can be put in small bowls of water, on small pieces of white paper or cloth, or on the appropriate gemstone.

On the Healer

The healer can use essential oils to open his or her energy channels. The choice of oil is an entirely personal matter. Only you can say which is in tune with yourself. Oils can be chosen on the basis of their being in tune with your own energy field, or with the energy that uses you as a conduit. Choose one of the following methods:

- Put a drop of essential oil on two small pieces of white adhesive paper and attach them to the soles of your shoes, under the center of the soles of your feet.
- Use the spray method, as described above, but on the feet.
- Put a small smear of essential oil on each foot, at the uppermost point of the inner bend or arch of the foot (underside of the metatarsal bone). This will have an effect along the whole spine, and on the chakras, and will help to clear your energetic field.

ESSENTIAL OILS AND DISTANT HEALING

Distant healing involves a person or persons transmitting healing thoughts to the receiving person, who is a distance away, perhaps many miles or even on another continent. The recipient may or may not be aware that healing prayers are taking place on their behalf. It is sometimes called "absent healing" because the person receiving the healing is absent from the room in which healing is instigated.

We are not talking about auric fields or energetic bodies but about the huge cosmic space of the universe. It's known that people on opposite sides of the world can think of each other simultaneously. Friends are often known to telephone one another at the very same moment — a real mystery, indeed. Thoughts seem to have no boundary. To thoughts, distance is irrelevant.

Whatever mechanism is involved in absent healing, and whatever space lies between sender and recipient, thoughts negotiate a way through all the invisible energies that now fill the airwaves, beaming down from satellites and aimed at us from radio and TV transmitters. The modern atmosphere is full of invisible informational traffic, like people's cellular telephone conversations, which might not be entirely full of love and light. Aside from this, we have all manner of rays coming out at us from computers and microwaves, which further clutter the natural energetic environment through which, no doubt, our ancestors also sent each other their mental messages.

Because vibration attaches to vibration, the single most important thing to send is love. It may be the most important element of absent healing, giving the recipient the support and strength necessary to resolve his or her own troubles and problems.

The methods to choose for absent healing are the spray or diffuser methods. Only very small amounts are needed, around three to four drops. If you feel that cleansing is important, use the spray method with salt. This clears the atmosphere of elements that may impede thought forms traveling. In a spray mister, dissolve half a teaspoon of salt in 250 milliliters of warm water. Swish the water around, then add three to four drops of essential oil and shake. Spray high into the air, trying to avoid letting the droplets fall on polished wood surfaces and other easily stained materials.

As you spray, imagine the water and essential oil molecules clearing a path for loving thoughts and beautiful healing energy, creating a time or space tunnel that charges through the air, or the land, or the ocean, to the destination of your healing thoughts.

Distant healing may have nothing to do with distance or space, but concentration is certainly needed to actually send the message. Essential oils can give light and clarity to the process of bringing the person into your mind and thoughts.

The essential oils can be used in a diffuser in the room while the distant healing is being projected. The lighter vibratory oils appear to be more suitable for distant healing than those with heavier elements, that is, those with a heavy, pungent aroma. Beyond this, you need to consider whether your healing intention is more concerned with a physical, emotional, or spiritual need, and choose oils appropriately. If you are sending healing for a specific condition, choose an essential oil that amplifies the healing energy being sent with its corresponding specific healing frequency.

Thought forms and healing prayers seem to travel very well on the light particles of fragrance that transmit love across the universe. The higher vibratory essential oils would be good choices to start with:

- Rose bulgar, for universal love of the heart
- Neroli, for the light that shines within it
- Chamomile Roman, a humble flower that heals the spiritual connections

If you send healing for a particular illness, disease, or disorder, and you'd like to use an essential oil that has healing qualities in relation to it, choose an essential oil by referencing the Physical Healing section in the profiles in chapter 11, and add that to one of the above three.

Healing Lists

Quite often, when people discover there is a "healing list" operating some-where, they think of someone in need and ask for them to be put on the list. The person to receive the healing may know nothing about it, or may hear about it months later when they're told, "Oh, I put your name down on such and such a list." It is always possible that the recipient may not want to be put on a list, or have strangers aware of the details of the ailment. Perhaps people should be asked whether they want to be added to a list before placing them there.

It is very difficult, if not impossible, to use essential oils with healing lists that involve more than a couple of people. The essential oils have to be chosen indi-vidually, taking several things into consideration, and if too much decision mak-ing is necessary, it detracts from the focus of sending love and healing energy.

ESSENTIAL OILS AND REIKI

The word *Reiki* comes from the Japanese words *rei,* meaning "universal," and *ki,* meaning "life energy," and refers to the universal life energy that heals and brings the body into balance. Discovered by Dr. Mikao Usui in the early 1900s, Reiki is a system of energy-activating attunements — using nontactile hand movements and symbols — that unlock a person's ability to use the Reiki power, either on themselves or on another person.

Reiki is said to have its roots in ancient Tibet, although its "home" is said to be Japan, and it's generally thought of as a Japanese system. For this reason, it might be appropriate to use Reiki with two Japanese essential oils: hinoki "cypress," or pine; and yuzu, which comes from the rind of a citrus fruit. Reiki was received while in deep contemplation on a mountain outside Kyoto, sur-rounded by magnificent pine trees, which are deeply embedded in Japanese spiritual thought, and inspirational to it. The smoke of the burning wood from these trees is used in many traditional Shinto ceremonies, such as for cleansing. Hinoki essential oil has a woody, turpentine aroma. Using it while performing the Reiki healing attunements or studying the special healing symbols might help form an energetic link to the original Reiki energy and thought form, which could be useful not only to the healer but to the energy itself.

The yuzu tree was introduced to Japan from China more than a thousand years ago. This hardy citrus tree, which grows up to fifteen feet, can thrive in surprisingly cold weather. It produces a yellow-green fruit, with a thick, pithy skin, that is used to produce the tree's essential oil. The oil is light and refreshing and universally liked.

The combination of hinoki pine and yuzu essential oils, in low volume in a diffuser, provide a good subtle energy environment for Reiki practice. If you wish to explore the deeper energetic history of Reiki, you might like to try using juniper essential oil, as juniper is the quintessential spiritual plant of Tibet, said to be where the Reiki energy was first awakened in humankind.

The above suggestions may be particularly useful when there are two or three practitioners working on a client at the same time, because all would have to be consulted and agree on any essential oils planned for use. A hinoki and yuzu combination might appeal to all.

For Reiki, use essential oils:

- In a diffuser — one or two drops
- In a water spray
- In water to wash the hands
- In water to wash the feet

Spraying the room with hinoki or another pine or cypress essential oil diluted in water changes the ionic balance in the room to a more positive (that is, negative ion) one. If the client is Japanese, hinoki will immediately be a reminder of home.

At the entrance to Shinto temples all over Japan, there's a special water trough where a person can wash before entering the grounds. There's a large ladle from which water is poured down over the hands, and some also ladle the water over their feet, or drop water from the ladle into their mouths, then rinse their mouths and spit the water out. Finally, shaking the ladle under the water, they rinse any energies off.

Such washing rituals can be adopted with essential oil use and used as a preliminary ritual to Reiki practice. Put a couple of drops of essential oil in a bowl of water, swish it around, and use a ladle to pour the water, spoon by spoon, over the hands, allowing the water to fall down over each one in turn.

ESSENTIAL OILS AND ENERGY WORKERS

No matter what type of energy work you do, it is particularly important to choose essential oils that are compatible with that type of work and that have the same vibrational energy as the energy worker. The physiological and psychological condition of the client should also be considered.

Essential oils can be incorporated into energy work in one of several ways:

- They can be diffused in the room.
- A drop of essential oil can be placed on the end of a smelling strip, which is then passed over the body in a pattern that mirrors the particular energy work being carried out. Do this before the energy work begins.
- Put one drop of essential oil on a small piece of white paper or cloth. Place it in the center of the palm of your hand, then cover it with the other hand. Rub your hands together lightly, then discard the paper.
- Apply one drop on a fingertip and spread it over all your fingertips.
- Apply one drop to any instruments used, such as a pendulum or crystal.
- Cut small paper circles and put one drop of essential oil on each. Place them at connection points, polarity points, energy points, or chakras, either on the body or on the clothes.

ESSENTIAL OILS AND CRYSTAL AND GEM THERAPY

Crystals hold energy and memory. They amplify or deamplify and can increase or decrease energy. No one knows how these mechanisms work, although there are plenty of scientists trying to find out. It's been said that the largest amount of information can be held on a ruby.

Crystals have an intriguing symmetry, being either cubic, rhombic, hexagonal, tetragonal, monoclinic, triclinic, or trigonal, reflecting the arrangement of the atoms or ions they are made of. All rocks are made up of crystals packed tightly together, but when there's a little space, crystals can grow and be seen visually. Granite is full of these little pockets of grown crystal, and it happens to be the rock that most holds radioactive energy. Perhaps this is why granite was used in the construction of many Neolithic dolmens, from Korea to France, because it causes interesting psychological effects. Dolmens are shelters made by standing two large, flat rectangular stones and adding another to the top to form a roof. The religious statues and walls of many ancient buildings were made of granite, including the inner surfaces of the King's Chamber in the Cheops pyramid in Egypt, where I spent a night and can testify that very strange visionary events can occur.

There is no doubt that ancient folk had a great deal of respect for the properties of crystals and gems. In Exodus 28:15–30, God gave detailed instructions for the making of a "breastplate of judgment," which had four rows of three gems set in gold. There are different versions of which gems were to be used and their arrangement, depending on which Bible you read. Below are three examples of differences in the relevant verses, 17–20:

THE BREASTPLATE OF JUDGMENT		
THE HOLY BIBLE — KING JAMES VERSION	THE HOLY SCRIPTURES ACCORDING TO THE MASORETIC TEXT	THE HOLY BIBLE — NEW INTERNATIONALIST VERSION
sardius topaz carbuncle	carnelian topaz smaragd	ruby topaz beryl
emerald sapphire diamond	carbuncle sapphire emerald	turquoise sapphire emerald
ligure agate amethyst	jacinth agate amethyst	jacinth agate amethyst
beryl onyx jasper	beryl onyx jasper	chrysolite onyx jasper

Details about the breastplate can be found at the Temple Institute Museum, in Jerusalem, from where I took the following information practically verbatim. When it was used, a piece of parchment would be tucked into the breastplate, upon which was written the ineffable name of God — Urim V Tumim. Each stone represented a letter, and as it drew down the spiritual energy from above, the related stone lit up. Only the high priest wore the breastplate and could decipher the code of the letters through a spiritual form of prophecy. The breastplate was consulted in decisions that couldn't be reached any other way by the king (David) or the high priest.

"John," channeled through Kevin Ryerson in volume one of Gurudas's *Gem Elixirs and Vibrational Healing*, is asked whether the breastplate emitted a brilliance. He said yes, the stones had auric properties and there was a blending with the priest's consciousness and aura, activating "a physical source of light merging with the auric and ethereal properties of the gemstones. This amplified the piezoelectric effect of the stones. . . . This effect was further amplified by the use of incense and essential oils with the breastplate." The piezoelectric effect is a very interesting property of life, affecting many things, including crystals, DNA, and the crystalline mineral apatite, which is found around collagen fibers in the bones and tissue. Basically, the piezoelectric effect occurs when pressure is exerted on the electrons of things, particularly crystalline substances, and electrical energy is produced. That pressure, or tension, can be provided by many things. Apparently, essential oils are one.

Exodus 28:21 says this about the naming of the stones: "And the stones shall be according to the names of the children of Israel, twelve, according to their names." The arrangement of these names is shown in a painting at the Temple Institute Museum, along with colors that presumably represent the gems, as follows:

Levi: smoky	*Simeon*: green	*Reuben*: red
Zebulun: clear	*Issachar*: violet	*Judah*: green
Gad: clear	*Naphtali*: pinky mauve	*Dan*: purple
Benjamin: opalish	*Josef*: black	*Asher*: bluish green

Apparently, only vessels made from stone were used at the ancient Temple in Jerusalem as stone does not transmit ritual impurity, which is called *tumah*. Metal and wood vessels were not used.

Working with gems and crystals is a very physical discipline, involving energies that are found in the rocks under our feet and in the cells of the human body. There are microtubules, for example, within the cytoplasm of cells and along the length of nerve axons. These packets of crystals move different chemicals up and down nerve axons, from the cell body to the synapses. How one crystal communicates energy and information to another is a scientific mystery, but it is a fact of physical life. The body also contains trace elements of minerals, such as gold and silver, which are, again, crystalline. Gems and crystals may also have an etheric body, and energy interactions, that happen in addition to the known properties, which are themselves amazing.

Crystals and many other gems are changed in color, depending on the minerals they have absorbed. Amethyst, for example, has absorbed iron. Color thus tells us something about the history of the stone, and about its mineral makeup, factors that need to be taken into consideration when working with gems and crystals.

Some people who use essential oils in conjunction with gem and crystal therapy choose them on the basis of their *perceived* physical color: for example, rose essential oil with rose quartz and myrrh with the resinous amber. For those who wish to know the colors of essential oils, a complete chart follows. This cannot be a definitive chart because the colors of essential oils vary, not only between species, but within one species when they're grown and produced under different circumstances. The variables are: the season when grown; location; soil; altitude; and, most important, temperature and duration of distillation and pressure of the steam. For example, a plant distilled under high temperature and pressure in a short time may produce an essential oil with a color very different from one distilled from the same plant but with low heat and pressure over a longer time.

GENERAL GUIDELINES TO THE PHYSICAL COLORS OF ESSENTIAL OILS FOR USE WITH GEM THERAPY

Colorless		*Colorless with Slight Greenish Tint*
Angelica Seed	Elemi	
Aniseed	Eucalyptus Radiata	Cumin
Balsam Fir	Nutmeg	Rose Otto
Camphor	Ravensara	*Colorless with Slight Bluey Tinge*
Dill	Rosemary	
Colorless to Pale Yellow	*Pale Yellow*	Chamomile Roman
Basil (French)	Amyris	*Yellow*
Black Pepper	Basil	Bay
Cardamom	Birch (White)	Cananga
Clary Sage	Carrot Seed	Cassie
Coriander	Cedarwood	Celery Seed
Cypress	Clove	Cinnamon Leaf
Eucalyptus	Ginger	Galangal
Eucalyptus Lemon	Hinoki Pine	Gardenia
Fennel	Lime	Mandarin
Frankincense	*Litsea cubeba*	Manuka
Hyssop	Melissa	Opopanax
Juniper	Neroli	Orange
Lavender	Oregano	Ormenis Flower
Lemon Verbena	Petitgrain	(i.e., Chamomile Maroc)
Manuka	Star Anise	Spikenard
Marjoram	Ylang Ylang	Tonka Bean
Peppermint		Turmeric
Pine		Yuzu
Rosewood		
Sage		
Sandalwood		
Silver Fir		
Spearmint		
Tea Tree		

GENERAL GUIDELINES TO THE PHYSICAL COLORS OF ESSENTIAL OILS FOR USE WITH GEM THERAPY (CONT.)		
Pale Yellow to Pale Green	**Greenish Yellow**	**Green**
Cubeb	Bergamot	Angelica Root Inula
Galbanum	Geranium	Root Valerian
Grapefruit		Boronia Violet Leaf
Lemon		
Mimosa Leaf		**Green Tinge**
Palmarosa		Linden Blossom
Amber to Olive	**Brownish Green**	**Light Amber**
Mastic	Oakmoss	Buchu Pimento
Vetiver		Carnation Tuberose
Yellow to Light Amber	**Yellowish to Reddish Amber**	**Rich Amber**
Caraway Seed	Ambrette	Balsam de Myrrh
Cinnamon Leaf	Cistus	Peru Patchouli
Citronella	Styrax	Benzoin Rose Maroc
Helichrysum	Tagetes	Jasmine Thyme
Lemongrass	Thyme	Jasmine-Sambac Vanilla
Reddish Orange	**Deep Orange Reddish with Slight Greenish Tinge**	**Dark Blue**
Rose Maroc	Hyacinth	Chamomile German
	Narcissus	Yarrow

ESSENTIAL OILS AND CHANNELING

New Age stores are full of volumes purporting to be channeled from beings living in another dimension to the earth plane. These voices are said to come from "ascended masters," "angels," "guides," "spirit guides," and "beings from other planets" or "stars." Invariably, they bring messages of love, light, forgiveness, and understanding.

I was curious to know what these wise beings had to say about essential oils and, in particular, if they would all say more or less the same thing. This was treated as something of an experiment. All channelers were offered the same bottles of essential oils, which were not named, only numbered. The channelers, then, were responding to the exact same aroma, and did not have a verbal or written indication of what was in the bottle. Both they and I may have, from the aroma, known what some bottles contained, but as there were sixty-five oils in the set, there was plenty of scope for olfactory confusion — especially as some of those used are rather rare and little known by name, yet alone aroma. The essential oil was put on the end of a smelling strip, which some channelers chose to hold in their outstretched hands, or took to their noses. Channelers who use particular hand movements while channeling asked me to hold the strip under their noses. Sessions were recorded, to be later transcribed, and an observer was present to take notes of the order of events, to record any physical movements and indications made, and to ensure procedures were followed to maintain the anonymity of the oils.

The following are extracts of what six channelers from those I saw said about the same neroli essential oil when asked to comment on its spiritual properties:

Channeler A:

"It is one of moving through difficulty, a herb of transition from one state of awareness to another. You could use it in a catalytic way, as a carrier of consciousness from one state of frequency to another...Its color is much more radiant and clear than the previous ones that we have discussed, and it is tinged with a very electric clear white blue."

Channeler B:

"To be used with care because it will inflame the passions. The passions are not only when we are in embrace, but we also are angry."

Channeler C:

"This will bring the sense of learning, what you would term the acquisition of knowledge is carried within the atoms herein. The ability, capability of input, that the capability from this is to be divided into three factors: comprehension, assimilation, and the ability to, as it were, discard that which is of no importance to that particular incarnative quality. In the realms this is known as 'the heavenly touch.'"

Channeler D:

"This is a very light floral extract and we feel that this should be used on its own. It should not be mixed with any other of the extracts. It would then lose its subtlety."

Channeler E:

> "The distillation is fine, but there's something at one end — I'm not sure if it's the beginning or the end of the process where the energy goes a bit wonky... and should be in a recipe of three to four smells, aromas, or whatever."

Channeler F:

> "This is more subtle, calming. I feel a lot of peace."

Neroli is the essential oil distilled from the flowers of the orange tree. It is very expensive, and in shops is often sold already diluted in vegetable oil. Many of the "pure essential oils" of neroli are of inferior quality, and their aromas are dissimilar to the high-quality sample offered to the channelers. I cite neroli as an example in this section because it is, for the above-mentioned reasons, not an oil commonly recognized, while it is one of the most spiritually active essential oils in the set.

Some of the channelers were clearly deluding themselves, despite having a striking air of authority. Channeler B, for example, said neroli inflames the passions, which it does not do. There were conflicting opinions between channelers, such as with Channeler D, who said "it should not be mixed with any other of the extracts," and Channeler E, who said it "should be in a recipe of three to four aromas."

On the other hand, channelers could make some very impressive observations. Channeler A, for example, who provided information on sixty-three aromas, made only one comment about me, saying of an oil I have a particular liking for and affinity with (which of course she did not previously know): "For you, Valerie, this oil has a special personal significance, for we see that it is fully aligned with your aura."

Some of the channelers were "bringing through" the voices of beings who were supposed to have lived in particular historical times and locations. As there is a very long aromatic tradition, one would expect these beings to be familiar with the certain aromas regularly used during their time and place on earth, and I made a special point of offering such particular aromas in these cases. However, it often proved that these aromas did not click — that the being did not recognize the aroma specific to the culture of their former incarnation. One ascended master from biblical times, for example, did not recognize aromas we know from historical records he would have been familiar with. Even if the physical aroma did not reach this master, he should perhaps have been able to recognize it from its spiritual qualities.

It was made clear to the channeler before each session that I was not asking for information on the physical properties of the individual essential oils, yet much information came forward in this respect, particularly with channelers who used essential oils, and most of it was incorrect. All of this discussion was accompanied by an air of great wisdom and authority, sometimes by people who say they channel characters known from spiritual literature — whose "channeled" advice some gullible people might follow word for word.

In *The Meeting of Science and Spirit*, scientist and author John White says, "I estimate that perhaps nine out of ten channelers are 'bringing through' nothing more than a fabricated subpersonality of their own creation." I'd agree with this. A channeler, then, might, instead of guiding you on your spiritual journey, deflect you from the course of true knowledge. In terms of general guidance this is bad enough, but when the guidance involves essential oils, which have powerful physical qualities, it is better to seek further advice. My advice is to tread very carefully. A channeler might say, "Use this oil, herb, or homeopathic remedy," when it is ill suited to your needs, or say, "Don't use this oil," when that may be the very oil you need.

The experience of asking many channelers the exact same questions was, at times, worrying. At other times it was interesting because of the concepts that emerged, the different ways of looking at things. On a very few occasions, I came away wondering if I had, indeed, been listening to an ascended master. Clearly, when you're planning to visit a channeler for a personal consultation, great discrimination is required.

There's nothing new about people speaking in voices that are not like their usual day-to-day selves. It's been going on for millennia, not as channeling perhaps but as "oracle-giving," and even "prophecy." At least today's channelers say they are just that, a channeler, and do not claim to be the source of the information that breaks through — sometimes without any warning, or desire on the part of the speaker. In the past, some people who found themselves speaking in another voice may have deluded themselves, or others, that they themselves were of an essentially higher intelligence, or in some way chosen or special. Indeed, making the distinction between true and false prophets, or ascended masters, has been an issue since time began.

Essential oils do open the channels of communication, both with the higher self and with higher spiritual elements in the universe. Among those who work in channeling, the following essential oils have been found helpful to that process:

ESSENTIAL OILS FOR CHANNELING		
Angelica Seed	Frankincense	Petitgrain
Bay	Galbanum	Pimento Berry
Benzoin	Hyacinth	Pine
Carnation	Jasmine	Rose Maroc
Cedarwood	Linden Blossom	Sage
Chamomile Roman	Marjoram	Sandalwood
Champac	Mimosa	Spruce
Cypress	Myrtle	Tuberose
Fir	Narcissus	Violet Leaf
	Osmanthus	

ESSENTIAL OILS AND COLOR HEALING

Color is not static, it's dynamic. Color is changed by heat, oscillation, and chemical reaction. A red cabbage might be red, but it's turned green by sodium carbonate, and back again to red with vinegar. That's chemistry at work. The brown gas nitrogen dioxide becomes increasingly lighter when heated. When it's colorless, if the heat is turned down, it becomes brown again. The human eye can detect ten million shades of color, which is a dynamic of light, vibration, heat, and chemistry.

Essential oils are a complex blend of many natural chemical components, with some having a "contents list" of three hundred or more. Molecules have a vibration, an oscillation. And essential oils are often heated, by means of diffusers, warm water, or the human body. They are dynamic energetically, in just about every way you can think of, which means that when we try to ascertain their color, many variables need to be considered.

When we see color, through the deciphering equipment of the eye, we're registering the wavelengths produced by light. Red has the longest wavelength; blue and violet have the shortest. White light is produced by the blending of equal wavelengths. Wavelength is changed by heat, which is why gray metal, when increasingly heated, will change in color to red, then orange, then yellow, and then eventually to "white-hot," the hottest.

When we see the color of an object, we see the wavelength that has *not* been absorbed. Inula essential oil is green because it absorbs nearly all the colors of the light spectrum except green. The *reflection* of green is what we are seeing, not the absorption of it. Something that is yellow has absorbed blue light and reflects the mix of red and green; magenta absorbs green and reflects a mix of red and blue; cyan absorbs red light and reflects a mix of blue and green. In color terms, things are not as they seem!

The light from the sun has all the colors in it, which can be seen as a rainbow effect reflected on a wall or piece of white paper if you hold a prism, such as a clear water crystal, in the sunlight. The prism splits white light into its component parts, wavelengths; the refraction is what we see. Red light is reflected least, and violet the most.

Plants absorb minerals from the ground, and essential oils contain trace elements of them. The type and amount of trace mineral depends on the uptake of the different species and the particular growing environment. When burned, minerals give off different colors; for example, potassium compound creates a purple or lilac flame, sodium an orange flame, copper a green-blue flame, and lithium, a red. Heat agitates electrons, and they give off more light.

The man who discovered why the sky is blue, nineteenth-century scientist John Tyndale, also discovered that essential oils absorb infrared rays. Indeed, essential oils are extremely dynamic in terms of taking in and giving out infrared, and electricity, and in terms of light refraction, chemistry and vibration, and minerals — all of which depend on other factors, such as where the plant material was grown and distilled, under what conditions, and who has been handling them. As for color, that varies too. See the chart of plant and oil colors starting on page 182. The first essential oil on the list, for example, ambrette, might be yellowish or reddish amber, depending on growing and distilling conditions, but it's not certain what color it is when it's heated by the hands, the body, warm water, or a diffuser.

There is no one color to any one individual essential oil. This is very clear when looking at their etheric color or, for example, their aura pictures. The dynamic *physical* multicolor aspect of essential oils can be seen at home, if certain conditions are just right. Put a large white container full of warm water on a counter, in front of a window that is receiving a lot of sunlight. Put one or two drops of an essential oil on the surface of the water, and adjust your body position to see, on the surface of the water, ripples of color rather like those seen on a soap bubble or on an oily patch of water. Catching this effect is not easy and may require several attempts.

This effect is known as "light interference" and is the result of there being two light reflections, one from the top surface and one from the under surface of the essential oil. Where the light rays meet, there is an interference causing some colors to cancel each other out and others to combine into bands of color, known as "the rainbow effect." In the case of essential oils, each one produces different combinations and strengths of color and, even more surprising, different energy patterns that can be seen in the way the colors swirl and intertwine, fast or slow, moving inward or outward, toward each other or not. If you can catch the light at just the right angle, wonderful colors can be seen — gold, silver, blue, green, red, magenta, yellow, orange, and violet — in all different shades and hues, from the very deep to the lightest of translucent color.

This light print may be the true physical color of an individual essential oil, and it bears no obvious visible relation to the color of the oil when it's in a bottle, or drop. The etheric color of an essential oil, its "halo color," is also different from its aura picture colors, as revealed by the PIP moving video pictures. And although both are dynamic, each has a different energy-action "fingerprint"; each is dynamic in a different way. When we're considering what is "the color" of an essential oil, then, it's a difficult task because there are so many colors to choose from — even when considering just one essential oil!

Some color therapists, when using essential oils, consider the plant species that the essential oil is distilled from — the color of the flower it produces or the color of the plant part used. This information is provided in the following chart, and should be considered in view of light-wave absorption or reflection. The chart also includes information about the etheric color of essential oils, but if you're working with oils on a person, his or her color field must be taken into consideration. For example, if a person is suffering from a great deal of inflammation, a blue oil (containing azulene) is usually applied, and indeed blue absorbs red, the traditional color of inflammation. However, blue also absorbs green. A green oil, inula, will absorb blue and is useful for respiratory tract infections, which cause excessive mucus and dampness within the body, usually associated with blue. But green also absorbs small amounts of red, associated with warmth. You can begin to see how complex the subject of energetic color really is.

In the early 1980s I experimented with colored oils, producing combinations of essential oil, base oil, and natural pigment. To see how long they could retain their color in ideal storage conditions, I put away in a box a collection of these colored-oil bottles. I took them out recently, and they were almost as vibrant and colorful as the day they were made. I encountered some difficulty in finding natural and organic oil-soluble tints and dyes, but eventually it was done. The greater challenge was in marrying up the three components — essential oil, base vegetable oil, and color source — in terms of their compatibility with the physical condition of the person, or the condition of the chakra to be worked on. When working with people and creating colored oils, there are many things to consider.

Considerations include all aspects of the essential oil's color, as well as the color of the vegetable oil in which it is to be diluted. As these two components are blended, a new color may emerge. Any tint or dye should be from a natural organic source and have the same physical attributes as the essential oil. You can immediately see that if you use a colored oil to counteract inflammation, say, the tint or dye should come from a plant known by traditional herbalism or phytotherapy to also serve that purpose. Each of the three components could also be considered from the point of view of their effect on chakras, and the whole person — not only physically, but emotionally and spiritually. Although some people might think using colored oils an easy option, a science of aesthetics or even "instinct," to be used therapeutically it's a science that can only evolve from a very broad knowledge base.

For those who wish to experiment, the following color chart may help. The second column of the chart shows the color of the plant part used in making that particular essential oil, which could be grass, fruit, seeds, leaves, root, wood, bark, resin, flowers, or flowering tops. Most species have a flower, even if that is a tree cone or grass spikelet, and the third column shows the color of that flower. Next is the color of the essential oil, which is followed by the density of that color: the letter *C* indicates clearness or clarity; the letter *M* indicates that it is of medium density; and the letter *D* indicates that it is dense. The last column is the etheric color, and it's difficult to capture by means of a few short words, which cannot convey the dynamism of these colors, their aliveness, and their degree of sparkle.

THE COLORS OF ESSENTIAL-OIL PLANTS AND THEIR OILS, PHYSICAL AND ETHERIC

Essential Oil and Latin Name	Part Used: Color	Flower: Color	Oil: Color	Density	Etheric Color
Ambrette *Abelmoschus moschatus*	seeds: brown	red with yellow center	yellowish to reddish amber	M	red-orange into gold, tinged with green
Amyris *Amyris balsamifera*	wood chippings: tannish brown	white	pale yellow	C	light yellow, orange, green
Angelica Root *Angelica archangelica*	root: light green	greenish white	green-blue	M	deep green and gold
Angelica Seed *Angelica archangelica*	seeds: green	greenish white	colorless	C	light lime green with pink and gold
Aniseed *Pimpinella anisum*	seeds: light brown tan	creamy white with yellow tinge	colorless	C	yellow-blue-green
Balsam de Peru *Myroxylon balsamum*	leaves: green wood: brown	white	pale amber-orange	D	rich deep purple orange-gold
Basil *Ocimum basilicum*	leaves and flowering tops: light green	white	yellow to pale green to colorless	C	green-blue to violet-silver
Basil Linalol (French) *Ocimum basilicum*	leaves and flowering tops: light green	white	colorless to pale yellow	C	blue-violet; light silver magenta, deep gold
Bay *Pimento racemosa*	leaves: dark green	white with yellow tinge	dark orange	D	blueish-orange to red
Bay Laurel *Laurus nobilis*	leaves: dark green to mid-green	gray-white with yellow tinge	yellow with green tinge/orange	D	orange-blue-green-gold

Name	Part: color	Flower/plant color	Oil color	Density	Energy colors
Benzoin *Styrax benzoin dryander*	resin: milky, light yellow	white	rich amber	D	orange-red, deep amber gold with a little blue
Bergamot *Citrus aurantium bergamia*	fruit rind: deep yellow	white tinged with yellow	yellow to green	C	deep greens, blues, magenta to orange
Birch (White) *Betula alba*	young leaves: pale green	catkins: pale green turning to brown	pale yellow	M	red to deep orange, green, silver
Black Pepper *Piper nigrum*	berries: green/red/black	white	clear to slight green tinge	C	red-orange-blue-green-gold
Boronia (Absolute) *Boronia megastigma*	flowers	yellow tinged with red	deep green	D	yellow-red, light green swirls
Buchu *Barosma betulina*	leaves: olive green/bluish	white tinged with yellow	light amber	M	reddish orange-gold
Camphor (White) *Cinnamomum camphora*	bark: orange; twigs: light green/bluish; leaves: dark green	white; red berries	colorless	C	silver-blue, green, yellow
Cananga *Cananga odorata*	flowers	yellow-greenish	bright yellow	M	green, gold, orange
Caraway *Carum carvi*	seeds: light brown (sometimes green)	white/pink	light amber	C	deep yellow, amber, red to greenish-blue
Cardamom *Elettaria cardamomum*	pods: green	pink	pale yellow to colorless	C	green, blue, gold, pink, violet

Key: C = clearness or clarity; M = medium density; D = dense

THE COLORS OF ESSENTIAL-OIL PLANTS AND OILS, PHYSICAL AND ETHERIC (CONTINUED)

Essential Oil and Latin Name	Part Used: Color	Flower: Color	Oil: Color	Density	Etheric Color
Carnation (Absolute) *Dianthus caryophyllus*	flowers	pink	dark amber	D	rich pink-mauve, blue-gold-silver with green flecks
Carrot seed *Daucus carota*	seeds: light brown	white	yellow and amber to dark yellow	M	orange, yellow, red, light green
Cassie *Acacia farnesiana*	flowers	golden yellow	pale yellow	D	red-gold tinged with purple
Cedarwood *Cedrus atlantica*	wood chippings: dark pink/light tan	green cones	rich yellow	M	blue-green tinged with deep orange and purple
Celery Seed *Apium graveolens*	seeds: light brown	white	pale yellow to deep yellow-brown	M	green, yellow, orange
Chamomile German *Matricaria recutita*	flowers	white petals	deep dark blue-green	D	deep blue, gold-yellow, deep green
Chamomile Roman *Anthemis nobilis*	flowers	white	translucent blue to colorless	C	turquoise, bluish purple, green, gold, silver, white
Cinnamon Bark *Cinnamomum zeylanicum*	bark: orange/reddish brown	white	yellowish	D	red, orange, gold, magenta
Cinnamon Leaf *Cinnamomum zeylanicum*	leaves: dark green and slightly reddish underneath	white	deep orange-amber	M	red, green, orange, blue
Citronella *Cymbopogon nardus*	leaves: deep green	spikelets: brownish green	yellow-amber	M	tannish orange tinged red-yellow

Clary Sage *Salvia sclarea*	flowering tops and leaves: green	pinky mauve/blue	colorless to pale yellow with green tinge	C	deep blue, gold-yellow magenta
Clove (Bud) *Eugenia caryophyllata*	buds: red	pink-orange into yellow corolla	pale yellow to dark yellow	M	orange-red violet tinged with green and gold
Coriander *Coriandrum sativum*	seeds: light green	pinkish white	colorless	C	blue, white, green, yellow, magenta
Cubeb *Piper cubeba*	berries: green/red/pink	white	pale greenish yellow to colorless	C	yellow-green, blue-red
Cumin *Cuminum cyminum*	seeds: brown to black	white tinged with pink	colorless with greenish tinge	C	orange, pink, green, blue
Cypress *Cupressus sempervirens*	needles: light green twigs: light tan	nuts: light brown	pale yellow	M	orange, gold, deep green, red
Dill *Anethum graveolens*	seeds: light brown herb: green	yellow	colorless	C	light blue flashes with green and pink
Elemi *Canarium luzonicum*	wood resin: rich amber with slight greenish-gray tinge	white	colorless	C	bright orange reddish tinge into yellow green
Eucalyptus Citriodora *Eucalyptus citriodora*	leaves: deep olivy-green	white-yellow	pale yellow to colorless	C	blue, gold, red, orange, white
Eucalyptus Globulus *Eucalyptus globulus*	leaves: green to grayish-bluish	white, creamy	colorless	C	blue-green tinge, orange

Key: C = clearness or clarity; M = medium density; D = dense

THE COLORS OF ESSENTIAL-OIL PLANTS AND OILS, PHYSICAL AND ETHERIC (CONTINUED)

Essential Oil and Latin Name	Part Used: Color	Flower: Color	Oil: Color	Density	Etheric Color
Eucalyptus Radiata *Eucalyptus radiata*	leaves: green to silvery bluish	white, creamy	colorless	C	blue-green tinge, yellow
Fennel *Foeniculum vulgare*	seeds: light tannish green	yellow	colorless	C	yellow-green, light green-reddish
Fir Balsam *Abies balsamen*	oleoe resin: greeny-yellow	cones: medium green to light tan	colorless	C	lime green into gold and silver tinged with red
Frankincense *Boswellia carterii*	resin: light amber to dark amber	pale pink, deep in middle	pale yellow to colorless	C	silver-goldish /yellow turning into a silvery mauve-blue with deep blue
Galangal *Alpina officinauram*	root stock: deep amber	—	yellow	M	orange, blue-green
Galbanum *Ferula galbaniflua*	gum resin: clear	white creamy with yellow tinge	pale yellow to olive-green tinge	M	yellow, green, white, mauve-blue
Gardenia (Absolute) *Gardenia jasminoides*	flowers	white (waxy)	deep yellow	D	blue-mauve, purple, gold, pink
Geranium *Pelargonium graveolens*	leaves: mid-grass green	pink/mauve	green to greenish yellow	M	pink-green gold
Ginger *Zingiber officinale*	root stock: yellow	yellow-purple, white	pale yellow	C	rich blue-orange yellow tinged with green
Grapefruit *Citrus paradisi*	rind: bright deep yellow	creamy white (waxy)	mid-yellow	C	green violet, yellow-gold flakes, magenta

				M or D	
Helichrysum *Helichrysum angustifolium*	flowers and tops: silvery green	yellow	pale yellow to amber	D	red, orange, yellow, blue
Hinoki Pine *Chamaecyparis obtusa*	needles: green	cones: green-brown	colorless with yellow tinge	C	white, orange, mauve, silver, green
Hyacinth (Absolute) *Hyancinthus orientalis*	flowers	blue	deep orange, reddish greeny brown	D	deep purple, blue-green, deep gold
Hyssop *Hyssopus officinalis*	flowering tops and leaves: mid-green	blue-mauve	colorless to pale yellow with green tinge	C	blue-pink-gold, green-orange
Inula *Inula graveolens*	leaves: deep green roots: brownish green	yellow	green	D	green, blue, yellow, pink
Jasmine (Absolute) *Jasminum officinale*	flowers	white	mid-red, amber	D	gold, blue, pink, green, violet-silver
Jasmine Sambac *Jasminum sambac*	flowers	white	mid-red, amber	D	gold, blue, orange, green, violet
Juniper *Juniperus communis*	berries: green, deep indigo	green	colorless	C	silver, white, blue
Labdanum *Cistus ladaniferus*	gum resin: orange	white or yellow with maroon/splashes at center	deep orange-amber	D	purple, orange, silver-gold
Lavender *Lavendula angustifolia*	leaves: silver tops: green	purple, mauve, violet, lavender	colorless to pale yellow	C	silver-gold, blue-green
Lemon *Citrus limon*	fruit rind: light, bright yellow	white with green/ yellow tinges	sharp yellow	C	green-yellow, gold tinged with violet
Lemongrass *Cymbopogon citratus*	leaves: green to mid-yellow	spikelets; brownish green	dark yellow, amber to orange-red	D	purple, red, orange, green

Key: C = clearness or clarity; M = medium density; D = dense

THE COLORS OF ESSENTIAL-OIL PLANTS AND OILS, PHYSICAL AND ETHERIC (CONTINUED)

Essential Oil and Latin Name	Part Used: Color	Flower: Color	Oil: Color	Density	Etheric Color
Lemon Verbena *Lippia citriodora*	flowering tops and leaves: light lime green	white	pale yellow	C	green, blue, yellow
Lime *Citrus aurantifolia*	peel: dark lime green	white (waxy)	pale yellow	C	green, gold, blue, magenta
Linden Blossom (Absolute) *Tilia vulgaris*	flowers	creamy white–yellow	light amber, orange to green	D	blue-mauve, light opalescent silver
Litsea Cubeba *Litsea cubeba*	berries: green	white	pale yellow	C	green-yellow tinged with magenta orange
Mandarin *Citrus reticulata*	rind: bright orange	greeny white tinged slightly yellow	deep orangy yellow	M	blue to violet
Marjoram (Sweet) *Origanum majorana*	flowering tops	white	pale yellow to yellow	C	green, yellow-orange to amber-red
Mastic *Pistacia lentiscus*	resin: brown	—	amber to yellow	D	goldish-red, green-blue
Melissa *Melissa officinalis*	leaves: green	white	pale yellow	C	deep blue, orange, red, green-gold into light blue
Mimosa Leaf *Acacia decurrens*	leaves: green	bright yellow	pale yellow to pale green	D	gold, orange, greenish blue into deep amber
Myrrh *Commiphora myrrha*	resin: light brown	white	deep orange, orangish red, yellow	D	red-brown-orange with touches of blue, deep green

Myrtle *Myrtus communis*	leaves: deep green twigs: brown	white	pale yellow to dark yelow	M	green, gold-pink
Narcissus (Absolute) *Narcissus poeticus*	flowers	white-yellow tinged with red	pale orange to greenish, tinged with deep green	D	blue-purple, silver-gold, deep emerald green
Neroli *Citrus aurantium*	flowers	white with yellow tinge (waxy)	pale yellow	C	white-blue, purple, clear gold
Nutmeg *Myristica fragrans*	nut-seeds: brown/tan	yellow	colorless	C	red, orange, yellow, blue with green tinge, purple
Oakmoss *Evernia prunastri*	lichen: bright green	green	deep green-brown	D	deep orange-red and green
Opoponax *Commiphora erythraea*	resin: dark reddish brown	white	deep yellow	D	red to deep yellow, green
Orange *Citrus sinensis and C. aurantium*	peel: bright orange	white with yellow tinge (waxy)	deep yellow-orange	M	purple, gold, silver, white, gold
Oregano *Origanum vulgare*	flowering tops	pinky-mauve	pale yellow to amber	M	red, orange-gold yellow
Ormenis Flower *Ormenis multicaulis*	flowers	yellow-orange	pale translucent blue	M	orange-yellow with green tinge
Palmarosa *Cymbopogon martinii*	leaves: mid-green	spikelets: greenish with yellow tinge	deep yellow with olive tinge	M	magenta, green, dark yellow, pinkish

Key: C = clearness or clarity; M = medium density; D = dense

THE COLORS OF ESSENTIAL-OIL PLANTS AND OILS, PHYSICAL AND ETHERIC (CONTINUED)

Essential Oil and Latin Name	Part Used: Color	Flower: Color	Oil: Color	Density	Etheric Color
Patchouli *Pogostemon cablin*	leaves: green	purple, white	amber to dark orange-red	D	red-orange, violet tinged with purple-gold
Peppermint *Mentha piperita*	leaves: mid-green	pinky white	pale yellow to colorless	C	pinky-green, silvery blue
Petitgrain *Citrus aurantium* and *C. brigaradier*	leaves: dark green; small twigs: pale green; budding fruit: sharp bright green	white with yellow tinge (waxy)	pale yellow	C	greenish, yellow, orange
Pimento Berry *Pimenta officinalis*	berries: green	white with yellow tinge	orange to yellow	D	red, green, magenta-gold
Pine *Pinus sylvestris*	needles	cones: brown	colorless	C	green, silver, blue, yellow
Rose Maroc (Absolute) *Rosa centifolia*	flowers	reddish	reddish orange	D	emerald green tinged with magenta and gold
Rose Otto *Rosa damascena*	flowers	pink	colorless to pale yellow with slight bluish-green tinge	C	pink, green, blue, gold, silver
Rosemary *Rosmarinus officinalis*	leaves and flowering tops	blue to mauve	colorless to pale yellow	C	spring green, blue-silver
Rosewood *Aniba rosaeodora*	wood chippings: reddish	yellow	pale yellow to colorless	C	greeny orange, into bright red and magenta
Sage *Salvia officinalis*	leaves and flowering tops: silver-green	purple, mauve	pale yellow to colorless	C	yellow-green, orange

Plant	Part	Color	Oil color	Clarity	Aura colors
Sandalwood *Santalum album*	heartwood: light yellow-tan	pinky purple	pale yellow to colorless	C	orange, pink, purple, green
Silver Fir *Abies alba*	needles: mid-green	cones: light green turning brown	colorless to pale yellow	C	silvery blue-green with light white
Spearmint *Mentha spicata*	leaves: bright green	pink	pale yellow to colorless to green tinge	C	blue, green, yellow, silver
Spikenard *Nardostachys jatamansi*	root stock: light brown	pinky violet	deep orange to deep yellow	D	amber-gold, mauve-blue, rich magenta-white
Star Anise *Illicium verum*	seeds: brown	white	pale yellow	C	orange, amber-red, green
Storax (Styrax) *Liquidambar orientalis*	resin: brownish green	white	white-yellow amber	D	orange reddish gold with blue tinges
Tagetes *Tagetes minuta*	flowers	orange and red	dark orange	D	reddish dark brown with gold fringe
Tea Tree *Melaleuca alternifolia*	leaves: green	yellow with mauve tinge	pale yellow to colorless, opalescent tinge	C	yellow-green, reddish
Thyme *Thymus vulgaris*	flowering tops	pink to pale mauve	light reddish orange, yellow to dark yellow	D	reddish orange, blue to deep green, yellow
Tonka Bean *Dipteryx odorata*	beans: dark brown	purple	deep yellow	D	rich red, orange gold
Tuberose (Absolute) *Polianthes tuberosa*	flowers	creamy white	dark orange	D	deep blue-green, gold to deep yellow

Key: C = clearness or clarity; M = medium density; D = dense

THE COLORS OF ESSENTIAL-OIL PLANTS AND OILS, PHYSICAL AND ETHERIC (CONTINUED)

Essential Oil and Latin Name	Part Used: Color	Flower: Color	Oil: Color	Density	Etheric Color
Turmeric *Curcuma longa*	roots: yellow	yellow	deep yellow	D	deep orange, green, red, gold-yellow
Valerian *Valeriana officinalis*	roots: yellow to pale greenish	purple, white	green to brown	D	deep blue–green, gold
Vanilla *Vanilla planifolia*	beans: green, blackish brown	white	dark amber	D	orange, gold, green
Vetiver *Vetiveria zizanioides*	roots: whitish/brown	spikelets: green	dark greenish brown, orange-yellow	D	deep green-yellow with orange tinge, blue
Violet Leaf (Absolute) *Viola odorata*	leaves: light to dark green	purple, mauve, violet	very dark green	D	green, orange, yellow into purple-gold
Yarrow *Achillea millefolium*	leaves and flowers: dark green and white tinged with pink	white tinged with pink	blue	D	blue-mauve into silver, moving into gold
Ylang Ylang *Cananga odorata*	flowers	creamy yellow tinged pale pink or violet	pale yellow	M	gold, magenta, green, purple
Yuzu *Citrus junos*	rind: orange-yellow	white (waxy)	bright rich yellow	M	green, red, yellow-gold

Chapter 11

The Essential Oil
Spiritual Profiles

*When the soul approaches the mysteries; when it tries to rally to the great
spiritual principles, the perfumes are there.*
— Marguerite Maury, *Guide to Aromatherapy,
The Secret of Life and Youth*

THE USE OF FRAGRANCE in making the spiritual connection is one of the
most ancient and enduring human activities. In some cultures, fragrance
has also been used for what we might term "energetic healing," although for
most people in history, and still in many parts of the world today, there is
no separation between body and spirit, and thus all healing is "energetic" or
spiritual.

The following profiles include information not only about the spiritual
character and potential of each individual essential oil, but also about their
therapeutic properties as used in physical healing, and their benefits to the
mind and emotions. All three aspects of an essential oil could be considered, as
each person has their own holistic profile that includes physical, emotional, and
spiritual aspects.

Essential oils are about vivification, the process of being enlivened in the
spiritual sense. Each person is unique, however, and is touched by each essential oil in a different way. Just as we meet people with whom we are in harmony
and who enliven our soul, so too we can discover in the superabundance of
essential oils those that release our spiritual potential.

The section in the following profiles entitled Emotional Healing shows the
emotional qualities that the particular essential oil will help bring out in a person. The section Physical Healing contains the therapeutic properties of the oil,
a glossary for which can be found at the end of this chapter (page 289).

CAPTURING THE FRAGRANCE OF YOUR FAVORITE FLOWERS — WHAT TO DO IF YOU DON'T HAVE THE ESSENTIAL OILS

When using fragrance for spiritual purposes, we do not always have to use distilled essential oils, some of which can be expensive or difficult to find. The extraction method, called "maceration," captures the fragrance of aromatic plant material, especially petals, and can be done at home. It produces an oil that can be rubbed on the body or added to the bath.

Simply put as many fragrant petals as you can into an airtight container and cover them with a vegetable oil, such as almond. Leave the container as is for at least twenty-four hours, but preferably for a couple of days, then strain off the oil, keeping it in a clean jug or cup. Throw the old petals away, but keep the oil and add fresh petals to it. Leave it again for a couple of days. Repeat this process until the oil has taken on the strength of fragrance you like. Methods like this have been used since very ancient times, and basically involve the vegetable oil drawing out from the petals their fragrant molecules, the essential oils.

For spiritual use, it is the fragrance of aromatic plant material we use, and this comes from live plants, which are often available in our own gardens or in flower shops. The living plants or flowers can be brought into our homes, and their aroma inhaled. We can even visit flower shops specifically to inhale our favorite spiritual aroma. Flowers such as pinks (carnation), hyacinth, narcissus, and tuberose can easily be grown in the garden, or as potted plants inside the home.

Spiritual fragrances are all around us. We can break the rind of citrus fruits and inhale the fresh zest — the essential oil. We can find spices in our own food cabinets or pantries. And if we take a walk in a pine forest, we can stop to pick up some of the dark green needles, crush them between our hands, and inhale their delicious fragrance. Fragrance is a gift of heaven, there for us all to enjoy, anytime, anyplace, any way we can.

Amber
Pinus succinifera

*T*hrough the veil of time, through incarnation and incarnation of mankind, this fragrance has remained, until washed up upon a shore or found buried deep in the forest. Such a fragrance has the ability to take us to the beginning of time, to the beginning of forever.

It can assist us in knowing where we have been, and to complete the cycle of where we are going. If time is circular, then amber holds the key. What spirit cannot be enthralled with such knowledge, such wisdom?

As it is breathed in, it holds the mystery of the birth of the planet, the mystery of the universe, the start of the creation of life, the Garden of Eden, the clay that formed mankind, the walk of the giants, the mysteries of the prophets, the masters who came to earth. All have known this fragrance from the start of the world.

Physical Healing

calmative, analgesic, antispasmodic, expectorant, febrifuge

Emotional Healing

To encourage harmony, balance, inspiration, visions, and inner knowing.

Aroma

resinous, warm, smoky, with a faint citrus-floral undertone

Combines Well With

aniseed, benzoin, carnation, cedarwood, cistus, clove, cypress, frankincense, galbanum, geranium, hyacinth, lemon, myrrh, orange, pine, rose absolute, spruce, yuzu,

Angelica Root
Angelica archangelica

Encaptured within its powerful fragrance is the possibility to draw close to us those angelic forces that are receptive to our needs. It is the revealing sword of Michael cutting through pretense and falsehoods, bringing into the light those shadows we have denied within ourselves. Yet, in this disclosure, it has compassion and an understanding of all our failings and of our longing for spiritual completion.

Physical Healing

antispasmodic, expectorant, diuretic, depurative, emmenagogic

Special Care

Avoid during pregnancy.
*
Avoid using on the skin if exposed to sunlight or ultraviolet rays.

Emotional Healing

To encourage strength, stamina, comfort, focus, solidity, grounding, and inner visions.

Aroma

earthy, herby green, rich

Combines Well With

bergamot, eucalyptus, grapefruit, juniper, lemon, lemongrass, lime, orange, rosemary, vetiver

Angelica Seed
Angelica archangelica

*W*ith angelic virtues, its fragrance spreads to all around, and in so doing spreads the protectiveness of the Creator, and etherealness, the lightness of being imbued with the might of the heavens. With gracefulness, angelica seed gently persuades the spirit to partake in the feast of the universe. It can shelter the vulnerable from intrusions into their thoughts and prayers, while allowing the guardians to give their reassurance.

Physical Healing

carminative, digestive, diuretic, stomachic, depurative, general tonic

Special Care

Avoid during pregnancy.

*

Avoid using on the skin if exposed to sunlight or ultraviolet rays.

Emotional Healing

To encourage inspiration, creativity, focus, concentration, and inner vision.

Aroma

clear, spicy, peppery

Combines Well With

bergamot, cardamom, carnation, clary sage, coriander, fennel, geranium, hyacinth, jasmine, lemon, rose otto, sage

Aniseed
Pimpinella anisum

One night a plant *deva* dared the aniseed plant to be strong and defiant. It protested, and ever since has assisted those who insist they have no need for prayer and are unbelievers. In defiance of what they know deep inside themselves to be true, they travel life's highway saying they have no need for a deity, that they believe in nothing. Yet when aniseed is given, perhaps as a medicine to calm the nerves, something else takes place — a puzzlement, a conflict. It can be dismissed, or a step can be taken to examine it further. And if that one small step is taken, then aniseed has completed its task — to make the conscious mind aware, even if protesting, that there is a conductor of the universe, and we are all part of the same orchestration.

Physical Healing

antiseptic, antispasmodic, carminative, expectorant, stimulant, galactagogic

Special Care

Can cause irritation to sensitive skin.

Emotional Healing

To encourage upliftment, stimulation, fearlessness, harmony, balance, and to dispel timidity.

Aroma

typical of aniseed: spicy sweet

Combines Well With

bay, cinnamon, clove, fennel, frankincense, geranium, ginger, grapefruit, lemon, mandarin, myrrh, peppermint, spearmint

Balsam de Peru
Myroxylon balsamum

*T*his is a sweet aroma, soft like the innocence of a child, yet with an unconditional love and empathy that stems from an understanding of the human state of being. Its soft, warm fragrance fills the spaces that have remained cold, untouchable, and unreachable, allowing the opening up of the heart without recrimination, in trust, and without judgment.

When in sorrow, the fragrance travels into the psyche to give comfort and relief from pain. It softly embraces us, spreading its fragrance around us like a cloak of velvet, smooth to the touch and gentle to the heart, cushioning us against emotional storms that may impede our spiritual voyage.

Physical Healing

antiseptic, balsamic, expectorant, stimulant, pectoral, antitussive

Special Care

Can cause irritation to sensitive skin.

Emotional Healing

To encourage warmth, calm, comfort, peacefulness, and the feeling of being soothed.

Aroma

vanilla-like resin

Combines Well With

cardamom, cinnamon, clove, coriander, grapefruit, hyacinth, mandarin, orange, patchouli, petitgrain, rose absolute, sandalwood, tuberose, ylang ylang,

Basil
Ocimum basilicum

*B*asil allows enlightenment to be absorbed by the physical mind-body, acting as a conduit, grounding, at the same time as balancing subconscious thought and conscious reaction. It is, then, a fragrance of reality — the reality of physical existence and the reality of spiritual existence. It soars through all the realms, holding them together, allowing integration.

It is a fragrance that not only harmonizes the many aspects of the person, allowing the light of the spirit to be held within, where it can illuminate the soul, but also stimulates recognition of those many aspects. It uplifts, awakens, and clarifies, and in this respect is particularly useful for those who, through life's emotional circumstances, have become numbed to the wholeness of human existence.

For those who have lost themselves through constant sacrifice to others, basil offers an opening of the heart and a view of the universal whole.

Physical Healing

restorative, general stimulant, antispasmodic, emmenagogic, stomachic, digestive tonic, intestinal antiseptic, anti-infectious

Special Care

Avoid during pregnancy.

*

Can cause irritation to sensitive skin.

*

Not to be used undiluted in baths.

Emotional Healing

To encourage positivity, purposefulness, concentration, assertiveness, decisiveness, straightforwardness, trust, integrity, enthusiasm, clarity, cheerfulness, and strength.

Aroma

warm, rich, fiery, sharp, peppery, aniseed-like

Combines Well With

bergamot, black pepper, cedarwood, clary sage, coriander, cypress, fennel, geranium, ginger, grapefruit, jasmine, juniper, lemon, niaouli, orange, palmarosa, pine, rosemary, sage, tea tree, thyme linalol

In modern Greece, basil is venerated because it sprung up at the place where it is said St. Helen found the true cross of Jesus. It's also associated with St. Basil and much used during the Festival of St. Basil, on January 1.

*

Holy Basil (*Ocimum sanctum*) is known in India as *tulsi*. Sacred to Krishna and Vishnu, some say also to Shiva. It's thought to deter demons from coming near, and thus became the protective plant of the house and of the spirit of the family.

It's said that every good Hindu places a basil leaf on his or her chest when resting; also that basil, planted on a grave, will help the soul pass to heaven.

*

In Nepal, basil is said to hold the spirit of Lakshmi, consort of the god Vishnu.

Bay Laurel
Laurus nobilis

*T*his is the fragrance of victors and poets, who have each used imagination and inspiration to attain their goals. It encourages the gift of prophecy and creativity, able to go beyond the normal activities of the brain, and in so doing brings forth tales of the future and of destiny.

A scent fired by the sun, protective and preventive — preventing the hold of unwanted forces upon the spirit, and clearing the confusion away. This is a fragrance to use when the way ahead seems uncertain or fraught with danger, when impoverished thoughts fly silently through the night to disturb our dreams and our waking consciousness. It protects, yet gives inspiration in the darkest hours, when the mind interferes and tells us that all is lost in the challenge to conquer the shadows.

Physical Healing

antiseptic, analgesic, antineuralgic, anti-infectious, general stimulant

Special Care

Avoid during pregnancy.
*
Can cause irritation to sensitive skin.

Emotional Healing

To encourage confidence, fortitude, inspiration, protection, direction, and creativity.

Aroma

spicy, sweet, fresh, balsamic

Combines Well With

benzoin, bergamot, black pepper, cardamom, cinnamon, clove, coriander, cypress, frankincense, geranium, ginger, grapefruit, juniper, lavender, lemon, mandarin, orange, rosemary, ylang ylang

"...resisteth witchcraft very potently, as also all the evils old Saturn can do to the body of man, and they are not a few...neither witch nor devil, thunder nor lightning, will hurt a man in a place where a bay-tree is."
— *Culpepper's Complete Herbal*, 1649 (1826 edition)

*

In ancient Greek and Roman times, bay leaves were symbolic of great accomplishment, in sports as in literature. Thus, victors at the first and subsequent Olympic Games were crowned with bay leaves, and the term *poet laureate* persists today.

*

Clouds of burning bay leaves were inhaled by the oracle of Delphi to help induce her oracular powers of divination.

Benzoin
Styrax benzoin dryander

No matter what touches the spirit, the soul must be allowed to speak, to be able to penetrate to the core of being. How misunderstood is this deep resin, which is the holder of the energies and fire of the sunlight, a joyous gift of the universe. Persuasive and direct, it opens the heart and mind to receiving gifts that have been denied, allowing the spirit to receive from the soul, in feeling, in knowing, in just being.

Benzoin is a pathway to understanding when all is confusion. It assists in the choices that must be made with the heart, and the softness needed when all contact with the self has been lost, helping guide us home to that place within, the inner sanctum of the soul.

Benzoin tells us not to dismiss things that are difficult, the outcome to situations we may not want, but to hear the messages and be guided by them. Some things can be difficult to accept, but as the years advance, we may gain understanding of the teaching of our lessons. In this, benzoin gives us its shed tears to use for guidance in that understanding, and for peace, on the pathway to inner enlightenment.

Physical Healing

antiseptic, antidepressant, vulnerary, expectorant

Special Care

Avoid during pregnancy.
*
Can cause irritation to sensitive skin.

Emotional Healing

To encourage comfort, elevation, peace, determination, while being soothing, cushioning, and protective.

Aroma

warm, balsamic, chocolately vanilla

Combines Well With

bay, bergamot, black pepper, cardamom, coriander, frankincense, ginger, geranium, grapefruit, lemon, litsea cubeba, jasmine, nutmeg, orange, palmarosa, patchouli, rose absolute, sandalwood, ylang ylang

There are many types of benzoin, and wherever it occurs, it's used to produce a spiritually protective fragrance. For example, in Costa Rica *Styrax argenteum* is used as incense in churches, while in Brazil *Styrax camporum* is used; in Malaysia *Styrax tonkinense* is often mixed with myrrh or chocolate.

*

In Malaysia, benzoin is burned to deter bad spirits, especially during rice-cropping ceremonies.

*

In Java, fishermen burn benzoin before entering the dark coastal caves where shoals of fish gather.

*

In Mali, it is used by shamans to facilitate transformation into other life-forms.

*

In India, benzoin is used in Hindu worship; in China, in Taoist elixirs to prolong life span.

Bergamot
Citrus aurantium bergamia

*T*he high frequency of bergamot works well in the auric field and also in that area of the light field that is closest to the body. It is an amplifier of light energy, energizing and magnifying, opening the heart to cosmic joy.

Bergamot lightens the shadows of the mind, bringing illumination and laughter. With this, it brings eternal youth and happiness, even to those who have put aside their problems, ignoring them until they have become so overwhelming they feel they cannot ask for help.

Bergamot teaches that the help of the angelic realms is ever there; all we have to do is reach for it. We may cry inside, our hearts aching, but bergamot will lighten the heart and dispel self-criticism and blame.

To any soul, bergamot brings freshness and illumination, lifting us from stagnation, bringing an awareness that the light will rescue us and take us ever forward to the realms of peace and joy.

Physical Healing

antiseptic, antispasmodic, stomachic, antidepressant, calmative, febrifuge, vermifuge

Special Care

Avoid using on the skin if exposed to sunlight or ultraviolet rays.

Emotional Healing

To encourage concentration, confidence, balance, strength, joy, motivation, good cheer, harmony, and completeness.

Aroma

sweet, fruity, citrus with spicy-floral undertones

Combines Well With

all essential oils, including: black pepper, clary sage, cypress, frankincense, geranium, helichrysum, jasmine, lavender, mandarin, nutmeg, orange, ormenis flower, rosemary, sandalwood, vetiver, ylang ylang

Birch (White)
Betula alba

A high-spirited essence of instruction and advice. It is there for whenever a clear pathway is needed for communication. It is a protective spirit that guards and guides, clearing away thought pollution or debris that may be lingering in the mind. It can stop unwanted energies from being transferred into our environment, not unlike the wind clearing away clouds so the light can shine through.

If violation has occurred in any form, then this is the essential oil to use in a sacred space before using other more spiritually connecting fragrances. It is the celestial dust-cart, sweeping up the misdirected and misguided thought forms.

Physical Healing

antiseptic, diuretic, tonic

Special Care

Not to be used during pregnancy.

Emotional Healing

To encourage protection, focus, and concentration.

Aroma

balsamic, woody, green

Combines Well With

black pepper, cedarwood, cinnamon, clove, cypress, eucalyptus, frankincense, myrrh, myrtle, rosemary, thyme

Black Pepper
Piper nigrum

This fragrance is strength and fortitude, giving us the bravery to venture forth into places unknown and unseen, fearless in our progress, with no questions but instead a deep faith and certainty in the knowledge that we will be protected and guided every step of the way.

Strength is often needed: strength of spirit, to hold fast against adversity; ingenuity, to avoid making decisions that may not be in our best interest and that we intuitively know is not the road we wish to take; and the ability to hold fast to our dreams and aspirations when everyone around us is advising us in our choices.

Black pepper enables us to listen to the inner voice of inspiration and to take chances knowing that whatever happens, we alone have taken them.

Physical Healing

analgesic, antiseptic, expectorant, tonic, febrifuge, aphrodisiac, anticatarrhal, digestive, moderate rubefacient, diuretic

Special Care

Can cause irritation to sensitive skin.

*

Not to be used undiluted in baths.

Emotional Healing

To encourage fearlessness, strength, stamina, endurance, motivation, flexibility, and comfort.

Aroma

strong, warm, and peppery

Combines Well With

bergamot, clary sage, clove, coriander, fennel, frankincense, geranium, ginger, grapefruit, juniper, lavender, lemon, lemongrass, lime, mandarin, marjoram, myrrh, orange, palmarosa, rosemary, sage, sandalwood, tea tree, ylang ylang

There are more than 900 species of pepper, but only about ten are used in medicines.

Camphor (White)
Cinnamomum camphora

*N*o timidity surrounds camphor, a fragrance of the warrior angels. For freedom of the spirit and enlightenment, camphor protects the souls of men. It is not the sweetest-smelling fragrance belonging to the angelic world, yet camphor may be involved in our salvation.

With the might of the angelic realms and the heavens behind it, camphor brings cleansing and purification, and has done so for aeons. For longer than we can imagine, the camphor tree has been guarding the passages of life; it is a spiritual protector and guardian of rebirth.

Physical Healing	*Aroma*
analgesic, antispasmodic, antiseptic, carminative, tonic	camphaceous balsam

Special Care

Not to be used during pregnancy.

*

Can cause irritation to sensitive skin.

Combines Well With

black pepper, cardamom, lavender, lemon, marjoram, orange, peppermint, ravensara, rosemary, spearmint, tea tree, thyme, yarrow

Emotional Healing

To encourage upliftment, stimulation, and liberation.

Sometimes referred to as "borneol."

*

Native to Borneo and Sumatra, this resin has long been highly prized as an incense ingredient believed to keep away malevolent spirits.

*

Throughout Southeast Asia, the wood of the various camphor trees is used in temple building and in the making of religious icons. Many large Buddhas have been made from this wood.

Cardamom
Elettaria cardamomum

*S*weet cardamom, bringing the mysteries of the Orient, is a fragrance to stimulate the memories from the cycles of incarnation and the creativity and abundance emanating from our higher selves. Cardamom gives us wisdom when we are overburdened with responsibilities, when we need to tap into our generosity of spirit to allow our hearts to be open and expansive in order to be gracious in our dealings with others. Also, it gives encouragement as we step forward to offer a hand of friendship when we see that a person is in need.

Cardamom assists in stimulating the spiritual senses, awakening us to the bountiful in nature and to the beauty there is in seeing with our hearts the often-hidden virtues in all mankind.

Physical Healing

antiseptic, digestive stimulant, carminative, stomachic, diuretic, antispasmodic, expectorant

Emotional Healing

To encourage clarity, concentration, direction, motivation, straightforwardness, enthusiasm, confidence, and courage.

Aroma

fresh, sweet green, spicy, balsamic

Combines Well With

bay, bergamot, black pepper, cedarwood, cinnamon, clover, coriander, fennel, ginger, grapefruit, jasmine, lemon, lemongrass, litsea cubeba, mandarin, neroli, orange, palmarosa, patchouli, petitgrain, sandalwood, vetiver, ylang ylang,

"...the cardamom seeds illustrate the bifold structure of maya or veiling. Mystics of all faiths have affirmed this duality in every aspect of life, pointing to it as the source of all creative activity." — Omar Garrison, *Tantra*

Carnation (Absolute)
Dianthus caryophyllus

Carnation soothes the soul, rejoicing in the rebirth of the spirit. It allows long-forgotten memories to merge in a symphony of being, of oneness with the universe. Touching inner feelings buried through circumstances, it enables messages from the spirit to comfort and cajole. Such joy is held within the fragrance that even the shiest aspects of self can be brought forth into the sunlight, to rejoice in the glory of heaven. We do not need always to voice our needs and blessings, yet we may have a yearning to understand them.

Carnation allows us to luxuriate in the knowing of the experience. The uplifting experience of reaching higher realms brings untold gladness to the heart and soul.

Physical Healing

calmative, sedative, neuro tonic, soporific

Emotional Healing

To encourage self-worth, communication, creativity, independence, tenderness, cushioning, openness, and release.

Aroma

rich, floral, spicy, honey-clove

Combines Well With

bergamot, black pepper, cardamom, chamomile Roman, clary sage, clove, coriander, geranium, hyacinth, jasmine, lemon, neroli, orange, rose absolute, sandalwood ylang ylang, yuzu

Only very small amounts of absolute oil are used in blends, as these oils can be very strong.

*

Bay essential oil and synthetic aromatics such as eugenol, isoeugenol, and phenyl ethyl alcohol are sometimes used to adulterate carnation oil.

Cedarwood
Cedrus atlantica

$\mathscr{S}$teadiness is the message of the spirit of cedarwood. It is the spirit of integrity, of stability, of solidarity in all things. It has qualities that are often needed when the spirit is weakened by living too much, loving too hard, and being unable to forgive. It encourages the strength we need to continue on our pathway, and urges us to hold fast to our dreams, helping bring our hopes to reality.

It can bring understanding from a nonemotional standpoint, while allowing compassion to be ever-present. Its spirit has the energy to allow us to continue with a job or task that may seem distasteful to us, and it gives us the strength not to feel revengeful. Cedarwood is the spirit of the ancients, the vigor and might of the universe, its elders holding fast the earth while living through many incarnations of the human soul. It allows us to look into our past while looking forward to the future in strength of heart and wisdom, and with the security of love.

Physical Healing

antiseptic, tonic, antispasmodic, regenerative

Emotional Healing

To encourage strength, focus, balance, fortitude, persistence, confidence, protectiveness, and concentration.

Aroma

warm, sweet, soft, woody, balsamic

Combines Well With

bay, bergamot, cardamom, chamomile Roman, clary sage, cypress, fir, frankincense, geranium, grapefruit, juniper, lavender, marjoram, neroli, orange, palmarosa, petitgrain, pine, rosemary, sandalwood, ylang ylang

Several types of essential oil are distilled from other species of cedar, for example, *Juniperas virginiana* and *Cedrus libani* (Himalayan cedar).

"The trees of the Lord are full of sap; the cedars of Lebanon, which He hath planted."   — Psalms 104:16

*

"...in [India] a fire is kindled with twigs of the scared cedar, and the Dainyal or sibyl, with a cloth over her head, inhales the thick pungent smoke till she is seized with convulsions and falls senseless to the ground. Soon she rises and raises a shrill chant, which is caught up and loudly repeated by her audience."   — J. G. Frazer, *The Golden Bough*

*

Used by the ancient Egyptians for mummification and by other ancient cultures for sarcophagi and palace and temple building material. According to Dr. Christian Ratsch, "The cedar...played a central role in the Egyptian tree cult; since it arose from the god Osiris, it became a symbol of eternal return. For this reason, its wood, but especially its oil, was thought to contain magical powers which the proper magical formulae could call forth."

*

The Native American nations use cedar extensively, both for medicine and for spiritual purification. The Guarani, for example, hold the cedar as sacred, using both wood and oil in their shamanic practices, saying the sap is a part of eternity. Cedar was the first tree their god, Nanderuvuzu, created, and it still stands in their paradise.

Chamomile German
Matricaria recutita

When used with purpose and direction, the fragrance of the blue chamomile assists us in seeking spiritual understanding. Its petals open with the sun, and it pulls down the energy from the heavens and solar system. When inhaled with purpose, it can allow a deeper knowledge of the working of the universe and of certain angelic orders who work close to the earth. When confusion seems to become prevalent in a person's spiritual life, and the laws of the Creator seem to have no meaning to the life we live on earth, then the fragrance can often help us understand. As we all already know the answers, it is just that we need a stillness to react to the wisdom stemming from God, found by meditation. It can help the transference of prayers, and gives clearer understanding of God's work, energies, and laws.

Physical Healing

calmative, analgesic, antispasmodic, febrifuge, anti-inflammatory, immunostimulant, emmenagogic, digestive, hepatic, vulnerary

Emotional Healing

To encourage communication, relaxation, understanding, organization, empathy, patience, and calm, and to soothe.

Aroma

sweet, strawlike, and herby

Combines Well With

bergamot, chamomile Roman, clary sage, cypress, frankincense, geranium, grapefruit, lavender, lemon, marjoram, niaouli, pine, ravensara, rosemary, tea tree

Chamomile Roman
Anthemis nobilis

*H*armonizing, peaceful, and soothing to the spirit, chamomile Roman resonates beyond the auric and beyond the seven rays. It operates in the realm of light and connects with the light body.

It connects with the inner child in us, allowing us to come closer to the spiritual realms for comfort and uniting.

Chamomile Roman is used for gentleness, when the spirit is sad.

The petals open their arms in prayer as the sun rises, giving thanks to the Creator, sending their fragrance into the heavens, where angels capture each tiny molecule and hold it close to their heart — to send back to the children of the earth in times of need.

Physical Healing

analgesic, antispasmodic, calmative, antiseptic, antibiotic, anti-inflammatory, anti-infectious, vulnerary, immunostimulant, sedative, antineuralgic, nervine, antidepressant

Emotional Healing

To encourage stillness, calmness, softness, gentleness, relaxation, serenity, spiritual awareness, emotional stability, inner peace, understanding, and cooperation.

Aroma

fruity, sweet, fresh, herbaceous, rather applelike

Combines Well With

clary sage, geranium, grapefruit, jasmine, lavender, lemon, neroli, rose otto

Chamomile Roman (*continued*)

"*Chamomile anthemis palaestina* has scented aromatic leaves and white, downy flowers . . . would very likely have been growing around and about our Lord's feet as He was speaking."   —W. E. Shewell-Cooper,
Plants, Flowers, and Herbs of the Bible

*

In preparation for passing to spirit, a variety of chamomile was used on the body of Rameses II in 1224 BCE — possibly as a scented oil.

In Tutankhamen's tomb, ten statues of the gods were garlanded with leaves and flowers, including mayweed, a type of chamomile, whose Latin name is *Anthemis pseudocotula*.

Cinnamon
Cinnamomum zeylanicum

ℒove, in all its many guises, speaks through cinnamon, to touch those hidden areas of the self that we have denied love access to.

Bringing into our hearts the ever-understanding love and oneness invites love from higher realms. But feeling that first, inner love is often difficult in the human state of being. The warm glow of cinnamon radiates through all space and time, transforming sorrow into happiness. It brings the realization that love is always there, if we tune into its warm vibration.

Physical Healing

anti-infectious, antiseptic, analgesic, stimulant, antispasmodic, emmenagogic

Special Care

Not to be used during pregnancy.

*

Can cause irritation to sensitive skin.

Emotional Healing

To encourage invigoration, benevolence, strength, energy, confidence, motivation, and generosity.

Aroma

warm, spicy, sweet

Combines Well With

bay, benzoin, cardamom, carnation, clove, coriander, geranium, ginger, grapefruit, lemon, lemongrass, mandarin, nutmeg, orange, patchouli, petitgrain, rose absolute, ylang ylang, yuzu

Cinnamon (*continued*)

Cinnamon has been recorded as being used in China in 2700 BCE, and was known to the Egyptians by 1500 BCE. According to Lise Mannishe, a papyrus recording the offerings made by Rameses III to the god Amun amounted to "one whole log, 246 measures and 82 bundles."

*

In Exodus 16, after being in the wilderness of Shur for three days without water, Moses and the people of Israel arrived at Marah, but the waters were "bitter" and undrinkable. Moses appealed to God: ". . . and the Lord shewed him a tree, which when he had cast into the waters, the waters were made sweet." As only date palms grew there, Dr. de Waal, in his book *Medicinal Herbs in the Bible*, has suggested that Moses used cinnamon bark. Two hundred fifty shekels of "sweet cinnamon" were included in the holy anointing oil, in Exodus 30:23.

Clary Sage
Salvia sclarea

The abundance within this fragrance is captivating, full of prosperity of the spirit. It has benefits for both the physical and psychological aspects of mankind, while also promoting contentment in a loving heart. Clary sage teaches us to be satisfied with our achievements, and brings the realization that most of our problems exist in the imagination and that issues that affect us will be resolved eventually. Clary sage whispers to us: be at ease and focus on contacting the inner spirit.

Clary sage carries spiritual timelessness within itself — a second could be a year, a year could be a second — and brings the realization that it's how much love we can pour into a second that counts.

Physical Healing

antiseptic, calmative, tonic, emmenagogic, anti-infectious, nervine

Emotional Healing

To encourage calm, confidence, grounding, regeneration, tranquility, revitalization, balance, and restoration.

Aroma

nutty, warm, light, musky, herbaceous

Combines Well With

bay, bergamot, black pepper, coriander, cypress, geranium, grapefruit, jasmine, juniper, lavender, lemon, lime, mandarin, patchouli, rose absolute, sandalwood, tea tree

The Latin *salvia* originally signified "good health" and has come to mean wisdom, as in "the sages."

Clove (Bud)
Eugenia caryophyllata

𝒮tirring the spirit, clove has no time for contemplation, only for action. Such is the message of clove: move forward, make things happen, achieve as much as your spirit can, without harming another. This is sometimes the most difficult aspect of what we have to encounter — not hindering others on their journey, nor giving them pain, while moving ourselves forward.

Clove assists in the awakening of the senses and in our striving for completion and oneness. It passes to us the sensitive confidence we need to be unafraid. This fragrance discourages inhibiting thoughts and encourages progressive deeds, making it easier to ride the waves while weathering the storms.

Physical Healing

antiseptic, stimulant, analgesic, antineuralgic, antispasmodic, carminative, anti-infectious, tonic

Special Care

Not to be used during pregnancy.

*

Can cause irritation to sensitive skin.

Emotional Healing

To encourage stimulation, regeneration, inspiration, trust, and inner warmth.

Aroma

rich, warm, sweet, spicy

Combines Well With

bay, benzoin, chamomile Roman, clary sage, geranium, ginger, grapefruit, jasmine, lavender, lemon, mandarin, palmarosa, sandalwood, ylang ylang,

Some commentators have suggested that the "onycha" mentioned in the recipe for the holy "perfume" in Exodus 30:34 can be translated as "nail," and indicates the use of dried clove buds.

*

In parts of Central America, it is believed that clove will dispel the demons of disease.

Coriander
Coriandrum sativum

*I*ts fragrance is fresh, as if seeking new horizons. It's cool, it's hot, ever-changing, depending upon the receiver's mood. The seeds are sweet, the flowers delicate, like a lacy cloud atop a green field. Fragrant yet subtle is this plant, like its action upon the human spirit. Gentle and compassionate, it intertwines with the inner depths of the nature of man. For seekers who wish to experience all things, before they feel sure of themselves and of the future thoroughfare to their soul. Who can understand the changing heart better than our guides? How can we change, yet still be true to ourselves and not stray too far from the joy of being at one with the universe? In this fragrance lies the challenge of change, helping us to go forward, even if timidly, rather than stay behind ever wondering, "What if?"

Physical Healing

sedative, antispasmodic, carminative, stimulant, tonic, stomachic, depurative, regenerative

Emotional Healing

To encourage creativity, imagination, good memory, confidence, motivation, optimism, sincerity, expressiveness, and enthusiasm.

Aroma

sweet, warm, spicy

Combines Well With

amber, bergamot, black pepper, cardamom, cinnamon, clary sage, clove, cypress, frankincense, geranium, ginger, grapefruit, jasmine, lemon, neroli, nutmeg, orange, palmarosa, petitgrain, pine, ravensara, sandalwood, vetiver, ylang ylang,

"And the manna was as coriander seed, and the color thereof as the color of bdellium." — Numbers 11:7

*

Coriander seeds have been used for thousands of years. They were found in Tutankhamen's tomb.

Cypress
Cupressus sempervirens

Cypress is often associated with the passing of a soul into the deity's presence, bringing comfort to those left behind, who will continue to hold their loved ones in their hearts. Cypress has frequencies that are in transition between the physical and the spiritual, which is why it can be used to assist in the passing over of a spirit.

Cypress has the ability to connect strongly with human frequencies and thought forms. With great direction, cypress helps connection with the wisdom of the universe.

It empathizes with suffering, the energies that emanate from a life in sorrow. It offers strength and energetic protection to those who need protecting, and to those who are feeling vulnerable and insecure or have lost their purpose.

Cypress can be used for moving on.

Physical Healing

astringent, antispasmodic, antisudorific, diuretic, restorative, cicatrisive, vasoconstrictor, respiratory tonic, calmative

Emotional Healing

To encourage comfort, change, assertiveness, understanding, balance, stillness, confidence, inner peace, wisdom, stability, patience, trust, incorruptibility, willpower, and straightforwardness.

Aroma

woody, warm, slightly spicy

Combines Well With

bergamot, cedarwood, chamomile Roman, clary sage, eucalyptus, frankincense, geranium, juniper, lavender, lemon, lime, mandarin, marjoram, orange, pine, rosemary, sandalwood,

The cross of Jesus, and Noah's ark, are thought to have been made of cypress.

*

The ancient Egyptians used cypress to make coffins, while other ancient people used it in their funeral pyres. Cypress trees are often grown in Muslim graveyards.

*

The wood was used by goddess worshippers to make images.

Dill
Anethum graveolens

We can find devotion and love in the smallest thing because all of creation is an act of love. A flower or a seed shines with love. A tree or a meadow has love flowing through it in the energy of the plant life. The majesty of the rocks and mountains have the spirit of protection and strength. The smallest seed is a powerhouse of energy, whether spilling into the body of the world or existing within us. The fragrance of dill is so sweet one is reminded of the wonder in the world.

The joy of creation is encapsulated in dill, and the taking in of spiritual nourishment from the heavens, bringing closeness with the angelic realms. Dill reminds the human spirit that the body is fragile and indebted to the earth. With purity and optimism, dill shows a clear way to complete the tasks we undertake on our journey.

Physical Healing

antispasmodic, emmenogogic, stimulant, carminative, digestive

Emotional Healing

To encourage tenderness, transformation, harmony, soothing, calm, and cushioning.

Aroma

unique sweet, herby spice

Combines Well With

aniseed, bay, bergamot, cardamom, clove, coriander, fennel, geranium, ginger, juniper, lemon, mandarin, myrtle, nutmeg, orange, peppermint, pimento berry, spearmint

Elemi
Canarium luzonicum

*E*mptiness fills the mind, silence creeps softly over the heart, and stillness enters — for elemi is a fragrance of placidity, of the quiet need to hear our own soul speak from deep within.

Elemi awakens the knowing that is hushed in the waking dream of reality. It speaks to the inner being, lulling the quickened heart and mind, steadying us so that we can complete what we have begun. Wrapping us in a cloak of sympathy when our spirit is most in need of comfort, elemi is soothing, yet it is strong, supporting our humanity, offering strength, and yet too, the upliftment we need to reconnect all parts of our being — our mind, body, and spirit.

Physical Healing	*Aroma*
antiseptic, cicatrisive, expectorant, tonic	spicy, citrus, fresh balsam

Emotional Healing	*Combines Well With*
To encourage soothing, calm, stillness, contentment, compassion, and peace.	bay, benzoin, cinnamon, cistus, clove, frankincense, ginger, hyssop, lavender, lemon, lemongrass, marjoram, orange, ormenis flower, petitgrain, rosemary, sandalwood

One variety of elemi, *Canarium schweinfurthii*, known as African elemi or elemi of Uganda, is used as incense in African churches.

Eucalyptus Radiata
Eucalyptus radiata

*A*ncient hearts dance to the beat of the eucalyptus. Fully aware of the past, eucalyptus is yet a fragrance of newness, renewal, and the seeking of new horizons. The fortitude it gives lies in its long existence as one of the earth's early healers, and the experience of generations of others who have taken eucalyptus' healing gift, often when no other help could be found. We see with clear vision the power of healing, and the many levels upon which it occurs, and with a final whisper, eucalyptus awakens the spirit of our own healer within.

Eucalyptus is a precursor to the fragrances that exist on an angelic frequency, its role to encapsulate the spirit within the physical form.

Physical Healing	*Aroma*
antiseptic, anti-infectious, expectorant, pectoral, tonic	woody, camphoraceous, with faint peppermint undertone
Emotional Healing	*Combines Well With*
To encourage emotional balance, concentration, centering, and rationality.	basil, camphor, chamomile German, cypress, fir, frankincense, geranium, ginger, grapefruit, helichrysum, hyssop, juniper, lavender, lemon, myrtle, peppermint, pine, rosemary, tea tree, thyme linalol

Fennel (Sweet)
Foeniculum vulgare dulce

*A*lthough humble and unflamboyant, fennel is strong, resonating with the infinite energy of the aeons. With great fortitude and strength it brings the light of solution into the shadows of difficulty. Its extraordinary power boosts the spiritual, recharging and amplifying, so it floods into the physical and mental bodies. This subtle strength clears and purifies the auric field of people, and the environment beyond, giving protection from outside influences.

Fennel brings the infinite light within it into the hidden shadows that may surround us, allowing our spirit to expand and soar.

Physical Healing

carminative, galactagogic, depurative, diuretic, stimulant, antispasmodic, antiseptic, vermifuge

Emotional Healing

To encourage enlivenment, motivation, clarity, perseverance, reliability, and assertiveness.

Aroma

warm, sweet, aniseed-like, peppery

Combines Well With

bergamot, black pepper, cardamom, coriander, cypress, geranium, ginger, grapefruit, juniper, lavender, lemon, marjoram, peppermint, rosemary, sandalwood, spearmint, ylang ylang

Fir (White Spruce)
Abies alba

*T*he spirit of fir extends around the planet, encircling us in its wide enveloping arms of protection, bringing down the rainbow of heavenly lights that shine upon us.

Every soul knows the fragrance of fir, even if only in the ancient heritage of their bones, and spirit. The fragrance is in the collective soul — a family member we love to remember, who is always familiar.

As we inhale the aroma of the sparkling green needles, we remember deeply the heritage we have shared with the trees, the plants, the animals, the stars, and the heavens. With the clarity of mind and spirit given by this fragrance, we can know we are One.

Physical Healing	*Aroma*
antidepressant, expectorant, analgesic, antiseptic, tonic, stimulant	fruity pine

Emotional Healing	*Combines Well With*
To encourage protection, steadiness, grounding, harmony, compassion, clarity, achievement, strength, and inner unity.	basil, bergamot, birch, camphor, cedarwood, cypress, frankincense, geranium, hyssop, lavender, lemon, marjoram, myrtle, orange, peppermint, pine, rosemary, thyme, yuzu

"I will set in the desert the fir tree, and the pine, and the box tree together: That they may see, and know, and consider, and understand together, that the hand of the Lord hath done this...."

— Isaiah 41:19–20

*

"The beams of our house are cedar, and our rafters of fir."

— Solomon 1:17

Frankincense
Boswellia carterii

*T*his sweet protector of the heavens operates far beyond the auric field, in the light realms. It is adaptogenic — it will adapt to a person's spiritual state of being, like an ever-watchful older friend capable of offering support in a wide range of circumstances. But, like a vigilant parent, it will not let us go where we are not ready to go.

Holding the wisdom of the ages, it waits for what is asked of it, and can do all that may be required.

Watching, with infinite sight, if it encounters malevolent energies attached to a person, it has the authority and power to assist in the removal of all that is unwanted.

In cases of spiritual shock or loss, when the spirit can step out of the body, even for a brief moment, frankincense can gently ease us back to our earthly home.

Frankincense is elevating, spiritual, and meditative, and holds some of the wisdom of the universe, that which is manifested in the spiritual self.

Physical Healing

tonic, stimulant, expectorant, cicatrisive, pectoral, antidepressant, antiseptic

Emotional Healing

To induce feelings of emotional stability, enlightenment, protection, introspection, courage, resolution, fortitude, acceptance, and inspiration.

Aroma

warm, sweet, balsamic, spicy, incenselike

Combines Well With

bergamot, clary sage, coriander, cypress, geranium, grapefruit, lavender, lemon, mandarin, neroli, orange, palmarosa, patchouli, pine, rose absolute, rose otto, sandalwood, vetiver, ylang ylang

Frankincense (*continued*)

"And the Lord said unto Moses, Take unto thee sweet spices, stacte, and onycha, and galbanum; these sweet spices with pure frankincense: of each shall there be a like weight: And thou shalt make it a perfume, a confection after the art of the apothecary, tempered together, pure and holy."
— Exodus 30:34–35

*

Given to Jesus by one of the three wise men, on the occasion of his birth in Bethlehem.

*

Included in the incense used by Roman Catholic and Greek Orthodox churches.

*

Frankincense is sometimes called "olibanum."

Galbanum
Ferula galbaniflua

A sacrificial fragrance that allows for the shedding of old ideas and out-dated behavior and attitudes, resulting in total surrender to the Creator. It sheds light on life's purpose and on the inner self. It communicates with the deeper layers of self, allowing a gradual unfolding of truth for those who have been blinded by success and ambition, allowing a sense of balance within the spiritual and physical self.

This fragrance should always be used with caution for what it might unveil — sadness, wrongdoing, untruthfulness, and crimes against the soul. It should only be used by those who have already traveled a large part of their life's journey, and having perhaps settled in their ways, find an urgency for stronger beliefs and the wish to walk in the light.

Be aware, galbanum brings with it all knowledge — in all its many forms.

Physical Healing

antiseptic, antispasmodic, analgesic, emmenagogic, expectorant, cicatrisive

Emotional Healing

To encourage calm, stability, direction, concentration, fortitude, and focus.

Aroma

green-pepperish, with a green-woody, slightly balsamic edge

Combines Well With

amber, benzoin, cedarwood, chamomile maroc, cinnamon, clove, cypress, frankincense, geranium, grapefruit, hyacinth, lavender, lemon, lemongrass, linden blossom, myrrh, pine, rose absolute, spruce, tuberose, yuzu

(use only small amounts in blends)

Geranium
Pelargonium graveolens

Geranium resonates with Mother Earth. It signifies the archetypal energy of goddess culture, and encompasses the energy of the feminine, of reproduction, of birth and rebirth.

The frequency of geranium appears to allow energy to become matter, and also allows the dispersion of matter through the energetic field. It must always be used with the great respect transformational energies deserve.

When the spirit is hidden, like a frightened child, within, geranium offers its warm hand of comfort, opening our hearts and memories, and healing the pain.

Physical Healing

astringent, hemostatic, diuretic, antiseptic, antidepressant, regenerative, tonic, antispasmodic, anti-infectious

Emotional Healing

To encourage solace, adjustment, regeneration, balance, assurance, tranquillity, and steadiness, and the feeling of being cushioned, soothed, shielded, and mothered.

Aroma

flowery rose, sweet, soft, green

Combines Well With

benzoin, bergamot, black pepper, chamomile Roman, clary sage, clove, cypress, fennel, frankincense, ginger, grapefruit, jasmine, juniper, lavender, lemon, mandarin, orange, palmarosa, peppermint, rose absolute, rose otto, rosemary, sandalwood, ylang ylang

Ginger
Zingiber officinale

*G*inger is a fragrance of valor and courage. It brings assistance to the fainthearted and to the weak, giving a sense of being capable and strong enough to carry on regardless. With the courage encapsulated in ginger's fragrant breath, we can utter that one crucial word, or think that one crucial thought, that changes our direction and starts the walk along a new and brighter road.

With courage, we can summon the angelic realms when in need, or pray from the heart without worrying what expectations of us that may bring.

Ginger provides a tool to break out of spiritual apprehension that restricts our ability to be free, and soaring high.

Physical Healing

antiseptic, stimulant, analgesic, carminative, fortifying, expectorant

Special Care

Can cause irritation to sensitive skin.

Emotional Healing

To encourage warmth, empathy, courage, assurance, optimism, and liberation.

Aroma

characteristic of ginger

Combines Well With

bergamot, cedarwood, clove, coriander, eucalyptus, frankincense, geranium, grapefruit, jasmine, juniper, lemon, lime, mandarin, neroli, orange, palmarosa, patchouli, rose absolute, sandalwood, vetiver, ylang ylang,

In India, it is said that ginger awakens *agni*, "the inner fire of divinity and creativity."

Grapefruit
Citrus paradisi

$\mathscr{G}$rapefruit rouses the human spirit from slumber, giving it the impetus to pay attention to the guidance being given to mankind. Energizing and enlivening, it disallows the egocentricity of just living for the body without making connection with the spirit. It can thus reconnect mind, body, and soul.

While we pray, grapefruit awakens the mind, allowing our prayers to be sung from the inner chambers of the emotional heart with force and mindfulness. Its purpose is to help us connect not so much with the angelic realms but with the angelic within us. It reconnects the silken cords that may through genetic inheritance have become broken, allowing us to be completely in harmony so that when the spirit speaks, the body hears the message.

Physical Healing

tonic, digestive, depurative, antiseptic, anti-infectious, restorative

Emotional Healing

To encourage joy, positivity, confidence, attunement, alertness, generosity, spontaneity, cooperation, and upliftment.

Aroma

warm, sweet, fresh citrus

Combines Well With

black pepper, clary sage, clove, cypress, eucalyptus, fennel, frankincense, geranium, ginger, juniper, lavender, mandarin, palmarosa, patchouli, peppermint, rosemary, thyme linalol, ylang ylang

Helichrysum
Helichrysum angustifolium

A fragrance of the devic world, helichrysum opens hearts to the unseen energies that affect our lives here on earth. It has a special purpose for "the walking wounded" — those who cannot reminisce for fear of the painful emotions that may be remembered. It is also for those who feel their physical self has lost touch with their soul.

Who will understand their pain? Who will understand why they feel shy and vulnerable when exposed, and only wish to protect themselves from the storm? Helichrysum's spiritual purpose is to make self-exposure safe. It cannot heal the past, nor protect the heart from future hurt.

Helichrysum allows a person to understand that to love truly also involves the acceptance of the pain of love — gladly, willingly, and without compromise.

Physical Healing

antispasmodic, analgesic, cicatrisive, expectorant, cholagogic, stimulant

Emotional Healing

To encourage calm, acceptance, dreams, patience, perseverance, inner strength, and awareness.

Aroma

powerful, fruity, fresh, strawlike

Combines Well With

bergamot, black pepper, cedarwood, chamomile German, clary sage, cypress, frankincense, geranium, grapefruit, juniper, lavender, lemon, mandarin, palmarosa, pine, rose absolute, rose otto, rosemary, sage, thyme linalol, vetiver, ylang ylang

Hyacinth (Absolute)
Hyacinthus orientalis

*C*arrying souls across the divide between heaven and earth is the task of hyacinth. Its fragrance sits so closely with the guardians that its heady fragrance drifts easily into the heavens with whatever spirit it must carry. Gentle and with compassion, the fragrance emanates from the flower's heads, which balance like ballerinas upon a strong stem. So it is with the spirit. As the time draws near for us to depart this earth, the fragrance connects us with the Divine deep within our soul. It becomes one with all that we are, and assists in the letting go of earthly ties.

In meditation, it has a quality unlike any other, heady and dizzy to the point of visions and prophecy.

Physical Healing

hypnotic, sedative, antidepressant, antiseptic

*

Used for aromapsychology.

Emotional Healing

To encourage calm, forgiveness, self-esteem, perseverance, equilibrium, trust, faith, and courage.

Aroma

powerful, hypnotic, green, deep, soft, floral

Combines Well With

bergamot, cypress, frankincense, geranium, grapefruit, lemon, litsea cubeba, neroli, orange, petitgrain, rose absolute, rose otto, sandalwood, ylang ylang

Only a small amount is used in a blend, diluted, as it is very strong.

*

Synthetics are sometimes sold as natural.

Hyssop
Hyssopus officinalis

$\mathscr{T}$his holy herb uplifts the spirit to the realms of divine wisdom, the source of creation, preparing the higher self for the final ascent into the heavens. It purifies and cleanses, awakening closed hearts and minds, bringing tolerance and understanding, unconditional love and acceptance, and the comprehension needed for the ultimate oneness with the universe.

A protective herb of the heavens, it is touched with the love and protection of the Divine. Hyssop is a quintessential cleanser, enabling a clarity of spirit, and recognition of the divine beneficent power in the universe.

Physical Healing

antiseptic, diuretic, emmenagogic, expectorant, antitussive, nervine, vulnerary

Special Care

Not to be used during pregnancy or by those with epilepsy.

*

Can cause irritation to sensitive skin.

Emotional Healing

To encourage awakening, acceptance, fulfillment, encouragement, leniency, direction, clarity, balance, and harmony.

Aroma

green, sweet, herby, spicy

Combines Well With

bergamot, cedarwood, clary sage, cypress, eucalyptus, frankincense, geranium, grapefruit, lavender, marjoram, myrrh, myrtle, orange, rosemary

Hyssop (*continued*)

"Sprinkle me, O Lord, with hyssop, and I shall be purified; wash me, and I shall be whiter than snow."

— *The Asperges Me*, said during
the anointing of the sick, Pre–Vatican II Roman rite

*

There are twelve references to hyssop in the Bible, most relating to cleansing rites, and there has been much discussion as to which species is being referred to. One of the most authoritative sources of information is the biblical landscape reserve in Israel, Neot Kedumim, near Jerusalem, and one of their publications says the following on the subject, quoting *Safra Metzora* (chapter 1:16): "The Sages were very strict in ensuring that only the true hyssop, *ezov* (*Origanum Maru* or *Marjorana syriaca*) be used in this ceremony 'and not *ezovion*' [in another version, Greek hyssop] 'and not blue hyssop and not Roman hyssop and not wild hyssop and not any other hyssop that has a descriptive name.'"

Jasmine (Absolute)
Jasminum officinale, J. grandiflorum, J. sambac

*J*asmine softly embraces the spirit and heart, bringing greater under-standing of the conscious mind and all its foibles. In its perfume, the wishes and desires of the heart are reflected and in gentleness we come to understand the subtle motives of the spirit. Our aspirations may not always be what is required to tread a spiritual path, and our wishes and dreams for others may deflect them from their path. Jasmine helps us to understand this, and accept.

It is said that jasmine has the ability to call the angelic realms close, and to be able to transmit our soul's joy and love to the universe, if the intent and purpose is carried from a clear and pure heart. In the world in which we live, space is often needed for a moment's reflection — to be able to consider the greater purpose, the master hand at work, and to inhale the glory of heaven. Paths trodden are often a mixture of joy and sorrow, but through it all we can survive; sometimes all it takes is another point of view.

Jasmine's purpose is to provide us with our personal haven, where we can find a greater conscious resonation with our higher self.

Physical Healing	*Aroma*
antidepressant, stimulant, antiseptic, antispasmodic, cicatrisive, sedative	sweet, rich, floral

Emotional Healing	*Combines Well With*
To encourage upliftment, optimism, openness, sensitivity, harmony, awareness, profundity, inspiration, and joy.	bay, benzoin, bergamot, clove, coriander, geranium, ginger, grapefruit, lemon, mandarin, neroli, orange, palmarosa, patchouli, petitgrain, rose absolute, rose otto, sandalwood, ylang ylang

Juniper
Juniperus communis

*J*uniper's message is to complete the tasks and learn the lessons. Meanwhile, it clears obstructions on our pathway to the divine spirit. While facilitating the transmission of our thoughts and prayers, it offers itself as a protective shield, disallowing impure thoughts to pervade our meditations and conversations with the universe.

A cleansing and purifying action takes place when juniper's fragrance is inhaled, and subtle changes are made — physically, mentally, and spiritually — as the unencumbered spirit can speak to the heart and mind.

Physical Healing

antiseptic, diuretic, emmenagogic, depurative, tonic

Special Care

Must be avoided during pregnancy.

*

Must not be used by those with kidney problems.

Emotional Healing

To encourage inner vision, upliftment, strength, vitality, sincerity, enlightenment, and humility.

Aroma

fresh, fruity, woody

Combines Well With

bergamot, cedarwood, clary sage, cypress, eucalyptus, fennel, frankincense, geranium, grapefruit, lavender, lemon, mandarin, pine, rosemary, sage, sandalwood, vetiver

"[Elijah] . . . came and sat down under a juniper tree: and he requested for himself that he might die; and said, It is enough; now, Oh Lord, take away my life; for I am not better than my fathers. And as he lay and slept under a juniper tree, behold, then an angel touched him, and said unto him, Arise and eat." — 1 Kings 19:4–5

*

The berries and twigs have been used in spiritual practice in many areas including North America, Europe, Egypt, Tibet, and China. Juniper is universally considered cleansing and purifying, and is often used in fumigation.

*

In parts of central Europe during the last three days of April, the smoke of burning juniper berries and twigs was used to cleanse the houses of evil influences, and juniper branches were fastened to the doorposts to deter such negative forces from entering.

*

To the ancient Germans, juniper was "the Tree of Life," and branches were buried with the dead to facilitate their easy passage to their heaven, Valhalla.

*

In Siberia, shamans have traditionally inhaled the smoke of juniper to facilitate trance and visions.

*

At dawn in Tibet, every household burns a fragrant wood, usually juniper, in their ceremonial roof stoves, known as *bsangs-thab*.

Labdanum (Rock Rose)
Cistus ladaniferus

*L*abdanum is a fragrance of prophecy, of visions, of quests in the search for truth.

It provides a vehicle to explore the knowing, and a means by which to acknowledge the existence of universal wisdom deep within. The emotions of mortal beings are touched by labdanum, and it can bring to the forefront of the mind access to the soul-level of all living things.

Labdanum cannot provide answers, nor can it speak, but it stimulates the eternal knowledge that is intrinsic to all human beings. There are no words to express this knowing, as no words can fully express feeling, but in the knowing we tap into the source of all creation, that which links us all.

Labdanum brings awareness that the universal spirit can be glimpsed and absorbed into our very being, although the complete merging with God must remain just out of reach while we fulfill our role here on the earth.

Physical Healing

antiseptic, antitussive, emmenagogic, tonic

Special Care

Not to be used during pregnancy.

*

Can cause irritation to sensitive skin.

Emotional Healing

To encourage visions, dreams, pacification, centering, joy, balance, and liberation.

Aroma

rich, musky, balsamic, herb

Combines Well With

bergamot, cedarwood, cypress, galbanum, hyacinth, jasmine, juniper, lavender, lemon, lime, nutmeg, orange, ormenis flower, patchouli, rose absolute, sandalwood, spearmint

"A caravan of Ishmaelites came from Gilead, with their camels bearing spicery and balm and labdanum, going to carry it down to Egypt."

— Genesis 37:25

*

"And their father Israel said . . . carry down the man a present, a little balm, and a little honey, spicery and labdanum. . . ."

— Genesis 43:11 (Masoretic text)

*

In the mountains of Crete, monks gather the sticky resin emanating from the stems and leaves of a similar variety of white and yellow flower, *Cistus creticus*, to make incense.

Lavender
Lavendula angustifolia, L. officinalis

*L*avender embodies the warm, protective love of Mother Earth. It is caring, cherishing, and nurturing, and energetically very active in the auric field, closest to the body, incorporating heavenly energies into the physical with great efficiency.

When deep sadnesses covers the spirit like a suffocating blanket, lavender gently lifts the weight. When the inner tears fall, lavender wipes them away. When depression clouds the psyche, lavender blows it asunder. And for those with worries that trouble the spirit, lavender lifts the veil of despair.

The mother of essential oils will not tolerate bitterness, malice, or jealousy in her mortal brood, and with compassion seeks to bring out the best in every one of us, letting us know that we are all her precious children, and we all have our destiny of goodness to fulfill.

Physical Healing

antiseptic, analgesic, cytophilactic, antispasmodic, tonic, cicatrisive, anti-inflammatory, restorative, calmative, sedative, anti-infectious

Emotional Healing

To encourage security, gentleness, compassion, reconciliation, vitality, clarity, comfort, acceptance, awareness, and emotional balance.

Aroma

fresh, herbaceous, floral

Combines Well With

angelica root, aniseed, bergamot, black pepper, camphor, cedarwood, chamomile German, chamomile Roman, clary sage, cypress, eucalyptus, geranium, grapefruit, juniper, lemon, lemongrass, mandarin, marjoram, palmarosa, peppermint, pine, ravensara, rosemary, tea tree, thyme linalol

It has been suggested that the "spikenard" of biblical reference may refer to the spike lavender, *Lavandula latifolia*, which grows in the Mediterranean region, or even to *Lavandula dentata*, native to Afghanistan and Iran.

*

For hundreds of years lavender has been a favorite plant grown in the gardens of monasteries.

Lemon
Citrus limon

 *L*emon clarifies everything through upliftment and focus. In this, there is centering and the impetus needed to send precious thoughts. Its fragrance enables our meditations to be deeper and our prayers to take flight.

The spiritual cleansing of lemon enables the entire psyche to react to the positivity in mortal as well as divine love.

Lemon represents the fruitfulness of the earth, and life, which is bittersweet.

Physical Healing	*Emotional Healing*
carminative, diuretic, antidepressant, stimulant, antiseptic, antispasmodic	To encourage clarity, direction, awareness, concentration, and liveliness.

Special Care	*Aroma*
Avoid using on the skin if exposed to sunlight or ultraviolet rays.	light, fresh, citrus

Special Care

Avoid using on the skin if exposed to sunlight or ultraviolet rays.

*

Can cause irritation to sensitive skin.

Aroma

light, fresh, citrus

Combines Well With

basil, bay, bergamot, dill, fennel, frankincense, geranium, hyssop, lavender, nutmeg, orange, peppermint, rosemary, ylang ylang

"And ye shall take you on the first day the fruit of the goodly trees . . ."
— Leviticus 23:40

*

The quote above refers to the four species that were directed to be taken to the temple in offering and gratitude for the gifts of the land during the Festival of Sukkot, the first of which is thought to be the citron, or *etrog* — *Citrus medica*. It is preferred that the citrus used in the modern ceremony have an elongated end.

Lemongrass
Cymbopogon citratus, C. flexuosus

In the quest to be free from desire and ego there can be no pretenses. This fragrance, powerful through its simplicity, has nothing to hide and could never pretend otherwise. It clears regrets or shame, encouraging forgiveness of those who have dishonored and discredited us. Plainly straightforward, the spirit of lemongrass illuminates what has been with the statement "Forgive, then forget." With the utter simplicity of truth, and in understanding gentleness, it reminds us that we are who we are, and that all life's experiences make the whole. With clarity we can see that the choices have been ours, and that freedom of choice is one of the many gifts the Creator has given us. Equally comes the realization that the outcome of following our spiritual journey will depend on the choices we make.

Physical Healing

antiseptic, carminative, nervine, tonic, calmative

Special Care

Avoid using on the skin if exposed to sunlight or ultraviolet rays.

*

Can cause irritation to sensitive skin.

Emotional Healing

To encourage upliftment, calm, balance, and integration.

Aroma

citrus, fresh, strawlike

Combines Well With

basil, bay, cardamom, cinnamon, clove, frankincense, geranium, hyssop, lavender, nutmeg, mandarin, orange, petitgrain, rosemary, spikenard, thyme, vetiver, yarrow

Linden Blossom (Absolute)

Tilia vulgaris

*L*ove in all its many guises speaks through linden blossom. It touches those hidden areas of self we may have denied love access to, bringing into our hearts the ever-understanding expression of love and oneness.

A graceful fragrance, it manifests a calm spirit, bringing a sense of relaxation to our prayers and meditations, and graciousness to all we do. A fragrance of mercy, it brings with it the ability to be merciful and non-judgmental in our dealings.

It may appear impossible, in the times we live, to achieve a state of graciousness, but this is within everyone's reach. The spirit of the linden tree is ever present in the fragrance, whether emanating from the flowers or in the aroma of its essence.

Linden can be used when things seem cold, and people unfeeling; when life appears to be rough, harsh, and uncaring; when the little niceties are gone, and it seems as if no one cares anymore. It brings back a sense of respect for others and the enchantment of being kind, and helps us to accept the kindness shown to us without expecting there to be ulterior motives for such actions.

Physical Healing

antispasmodic, antidepressant, nervine, tonic, calmative

Emotional Healing

To encourage relaxation, calm, self-confidence, security, balance, equilibrium, and the feeling of being soothed.

Aroma

light, floral, sweet

Combines Well With

black pepper, carnation, clove, frankincense, geranium, hyacinth, jasmine, lemon, mandarin, neroli, orange, petitgrain, rose absolute, rose otto, sandalwood, tuberose, ylang ylang

"There are references in more than one land to a Paradise among the mountains. It figures in the fairy stories of Central Europe . . . with its linden Tree of Immortality, the hiding place of a fairy lady, its dancing nymphs and its dwarfs; the king of dwarfs has a cloak of invisibility which he wraps around those mortals he carries away."
— Donald A. Mackenzie, *China and Japan: Myths and Legends*

*

The bark of the linden tree was once widely used, in woven form, as boat sails and clothing. Italian Renaissance paintings sometimes show the Virgin Mary wearing a skirt of linden bark.

*

Linden is often called "lime tree," although no limes grow from it.

Mandarin
Citrus reticulata, C. nobilis

The gentleness and sweetness of spirit is gathered in the arms of this fragrance. But however gentle it may be, there is a vigor and sprightliness in how mandarin stirs the spirit. At times, when we feel fully connected to the source of all creation, and still enough to hear the celestial music, we touch the spirit held within mandarin.

The elders gather where ancient fragrances play, and although mandarin is young, it still attracts the attention of the elders.

Mandarin can be inhaled whenever we feel the urge to make the connection with other realms and hear the music of the spheres.

Physical Healing	*Aroma*
tonic, calmative, antispasmodic, antiseptic	sweet, light, floral, fruity citrus
Emotional Healing	*Combines Well With*
To encourage calm, upliftment, inspiration, soothing, integrity, and tranquillity.	basil, black pepper, chamomile Roman, cinnamon clove, frankincense, geranium, grapefruit, jasmine, juniper, lemon, neroli, palmarosa, patchouli, petitgrain, rose otto, sandalwood, ylang ylang

Japanese myths regarding the "fruit of the everlasting fragrant tree" are quite likely referring to mandarin.

Marjoram (Sweet)
Origanum majorana

 arjoram calms the senses and allows peacefulness to come into a frantic world. It stills the mind long enough to allow the quiet voice within to communicate with the soul. Its warmth carries with it the fire and sparks of the cosmos, with which we can make a connection to our own internal fire. With its warmth comes a deeply centered peace that has flowed with the tide of humanity's evolution, holding within its fragrance all that humanity has borne.

Tread carefully, it tells us; speak not of evil or be judgmental, lest you too be judged. Try instead to forgive without judgment, without criticism, and for no other reason than to have a clear, untroubled heart.

Physical Healing

analgesic, antispasmodic, vasodilator, calmative, expectorant, digestive, vulnerary, antitussive, anti-infectious, emmenagogic

Emotional Healing

To encourage calm, balance, integrity, perseverance, and sincerity.

Aroma

warm, spicy, herbaceous

Combines Well With

basil, bergamot, black pepper, cedarwood, chamomile Roman, chamomile German, clary sage, cypress, eucalyptus citriodora, eucalyptus radiata, fennel, juniper, lavender, lemon, orange, peppermint, pine, rosemary, tea tree, thyme linalol

Marjoram (*continued*)

According to some sources, a species of marjoram, (*Origanum syriacum*), is the "hyssop" of biblical reference. It grows abundantly in the Holy Land, and as it has very hairy stems, would have been an appropriate plant to use as a "sprinkler" in the biblical context.

*

Marjoram is said to be the herb of the Egyptian god Sobek. Often used in the funerary garlands put around the heads of mummified bodies.

*

Used in unguents and perfumes in the ancient world since known records.

Melissa
Melissa officinalis

*M*elissa vibrates at a very high light frequency and travels very far. The energy it brings into the spirit comes from a place more distant than we can imagine, beyond the sun, beyond the stars. When the magnetic energy is at a low ebb, melissa supports our need with an understanding that defies words.

Melissa is a spiritual conduit and is thus a precious gift of the heavens at any time, but perhaps is especially appreciated before meditation or prayer.

Physical Healing

antiseptic, calmative, antidepressant, stimulant

Special Care

Can cause irritation to sensitive skin.

Emotional Healing

To encourage strength, revitalization, gentleness, peace, progressiveness, and cheerfulness.

Aroma

citrus, light, fresh

Combines Well With

chamomile Roman, frankincense, geranium, neroli, petitgrain, rose absolute, rose otto

(most often used on its own)

Myrrh
Commiphora myrrha

*T*his deep fragrance resonates with the wounded healer — the wounds running deep, carrying the pain of others — for infinity. The fragrance enables the letting go of the need to battle for the just against the unjust.

"The meaning of life," so often sought, has no meaning when the purpose of life is realized! This realization can come from deep within the heart after the emotional wounds have healed. Our spirit can also feel wounded, although it is always protected, but sometimes it seems outside our grasp. Myrrh, with all its submerged meanings, links with the pathway of the soul, standing at the very crossroads. It would be so easy to walk down any of the roads, hanging on to our wounds, but myrrh helps us to realize the need to let go, to forgive, and to move forward.

Physical Healing

pectoral, antiseptic, antispasmodic, cicatrisive, expectorant, astringent, vulnerary

Special Care

Not to be used during pregnancy.

Emotional Healing

To encourage fortitude, courage, peace, calm, sympathy, acceptance, and mastery.

Aroma

warm, slightly musty, earthy

Combines Well With

bergamot, chamomile German, cypress, eucalyptus citriodora, frankincense, galbanum, geranium, grapefruit, hyssop, juniper, lavender, lemon, palmarosa, patchouli, pine, rosemary, sandalwood, ylang ylang

"Moreover the Lord spake unto Moses, saying, Take thou also unto thee principal spices, of pure myrrh five hundred shekels. . . ."

— Exodus 30:22–23

*

". . . for so were the days of their purifications accomplished, to wit, six months with oil of myrrh, and six months with sweet odors, and with other things for the purifying of the women. . . ."

— Esther 2:12

*

"Who is this that cometh out of the wilderness like pillars of smoke, perfumed with myrrh and frankincense, with all powders of the merchant?"

— Solomon 3:6

*

Given as a gift to baby Jesus by one of the three wise men, at his birth in Bethlehem.

*

Used for more than four thousand years. The ancient Egyptians burned it at midday, in praise of the sun god Ra; they also used it in their *Kyphi* incense, and in embalming.

Myrtle
Myrtus communis

The fragrance of myrtle allows entrance to the pure and absolute, where ego has no entrance pass, where all is One and One becomes all, where there is no beginning or end. It tells of going forward carried within the spirit, reminding us that this existence is in preparation for another along the evolutionary cycle, which we shall transcend.

Its spirit is energetic truth, and forgiveness, giving support to the unsupported and teaching that divine love embraces all living beings.

Physical Healing	*Aroma*
antiseptic, expectorant, tonic, calmative	sweet, camphoraceous, herbaceous, green

Emotional Healing	*Combines Well With*
To encourage upliftment, comfort, forgiveness, acceptance, empowerment, and harmony.	basil, bay, benzoin, bergamot, cardamom, cinnamon, clove, eucalyptus, galbanum, geranium, ginger, helichrysum, lemon, mandarin, orange, rosemary

"And they answered the angel of the Lord that stood among the myrtle trees. . . ."

— Zechariah 1:11

*

". . . instead of the brier shall come up the myrtle tree: and it shall be to the Lord for a name, for an everlasting sign that shall not be cut off."

— Isaiah 55:13

*

"Go forth unto the mount, and fetch olive branches, and pine branches, and myrtle branches, and palm branches, and branches of thick trees, to make booths, as it is written."

— Nehemiah 8:15

*

The myrtle was a sign of immortality to the people living in the ancient Near East, perhaps because it remains fresh for several weeks after being cut. Known as *hadass* in Hebrew, myrtle is said to be the quintessential fragrant plant of Israel, and as such is incorporated into the spice box used on the Sabbath evening, wherever possible.

Narcissus (Absolute)
Narcissus poeticus

*N*arcissus is a key holder of the doorway to realms beyond inspiration and imagination, a fragrance on which to dream of things untold, unheard, and unseen by mortal beings, in the heavenly domain.

Protecting our fragility from fear and anguish, narcissus keeps us soaring into infinity, bypassing mortal conditions, linking us with the lore of worlds that have no beginning, nor end. Such is the effect upon the spirit of one who inhales narcissus with spiritual intent. It is not for the fainthearted, for no mortal can say where it may take you.

Narcissus can assist in overcoming the blockages we set on our pathway, and in attaining greater understanding of the unknown.

Physical Healing	*Aroma*
antispasmodic, sedative	heavy, green floral

Special Care	*Combines Well With*
Not to be used during pregnancy.	bois de rose, cinnamon, clove, grapefruit, ho-wood, hyacinth, jasmine, lemon, mandarin, orange, sandalwood, tuberose, ylang ylang
Emotional Healing	*(use only in small amounts; principal use as perfume or room fragrance)*
To encourage inspiration, creativity, stillness, and inner vision.	

According to Greek mythology, the soul of the flower-god, Narcissus, was captured by the Titans by means of a magic reflecting pool, the home of Echo and other water nymphs. With his soul entrapped, Narcissus died, but he reappeared as the spring flower named for him.

Neroli
Citrus aurantium, C. brigaradia, C. vulgaris

*N*eroli touches the realms of the angels, and anyone who uses it is brushed with the light of angels' wings. Neroli is one of the most precious essential oils, its vibration being one of the highest among them. It may be that it resonates with energy from another light-time in the universe, perhaps taking its light from another sun in the vast cosmos. Wherever its subtle and luminescent quality comes from, it is omnipresent.

Neroli is itself pure spirit, representing the purity in all things. It is always loving and peaceful. Neroli brings light into any day, but is especially useful whenever mistrust has overtaken reason, or during dark periods of deep depression.

Neroli has another purpose — to bring self-recognition and relief. Our pain and sorrow is sometimes brought about because we have not seen how we might have affected others and inadvertently caused a rift or hurt others. Neroli allows the reflection that can throw light on the wounds that tie us to old patterns of relating. As truth is revealed, the self emerges into wholeness and unconditional love, stirring the spirit in ways that can be both unexpected and liberating. Then, the spirit can really soar.

Physical Healing

antidepressant, anti-infectious, tonic, cytophilactic, calmative, cicatrisive

Emotional Healing

To encourage lightness, the lifting of sorrows, completeness, joy, understanding, calm, regeneration, and peace, and to feel guided.

Aroma

highly radiant, sweet, floral

Combines Well With

chamomile Roman, coriander, frankincense, geranium, grapefruit, jasmine, juniper, lavender, lemon, mandarin, orange, petitgrain, rose otto, sandalwood, ylang ylang, yuzu

Nutmeg
Myristica fragrans

𝒩utmeg brings hopes, dreams, and prayers to their rightful home, and in so doing, the highest elements of the ego take their place within spiritual wonderment. When the ego has received many life blows, is depressed, or unable to connect with the higher realms, nutmeg assists in the reconnection.

It is hard to see how our lives have affected others, and sometimes we might have brought pain and sorrow. When there is recognition, however, there is also relief. This opening of recognition is never accomplished without reflection and is seldom easy. But the wounds and ties that hold us fast can deter us from finding our true selves, and as self emerges into wholeness, then a stirring of the spirit occurs that is liberating, and at times unexpected, as it allows the spirit to soar.

Physical Healing	*Aroma*
analgesic, antiseptic, carminative, emmenogogic, tonic, nervine	spicy, light, warm, fresh
Special Care	*Combines Well With*
Not to be used during pregnancy.	bay, cinnamon, clove, geranium, jasmine, lemon, lime, orange, rose absolute
Emotional Healing	
To encourage calm, peace, visions, dreams, unity, comfort, and stillness.	*(use only in small amounts)*

Nutmeg is one of the oldest cultivated plants.

*

In Malaysia, nutmeg was given to people possessed by spirits, to drive them out.

*

In India, nutmeg was known as *mada shaunda*, the "narcotic fruit."

Orange
Citrus sinensis

*O*range is imbued with the energy of the sunlight and the radiance of the stars. Its fragrance has the adaptability required of such a high energy. So, at times it may be gentle, at other times it may give the determination needed to enliven the spiritual sense of being.

Orange contains the joy and magnificence of the light of the heavens. Bursting with vitality, it brings happiness to the heavyhearted and to those who seem lost. It brings newness and regeneration. It can rekindle a spark long forgotten and revitalize spiritual connections to a soul grown dim through living too hard, too fast, too painfully.

Orange conquers fears of letting go, and obsessions. The fragrance uplifts those with obsessions so they can see the full spectrum of light.

Physical Healing

calmative, sedative, stomachic, cholagogic, diuretic, tonic, antispasmodic, antiseptic, depurative

Emotional Healing

To encourage joy, upliftment, lightheartedness, regeneration, creativity, positivity, and self-confidence.

Aroma

fresh, fruity, tangy, sweet

Combines Well With

bay, benzoin, bergamot, black pepper, cinnamon, clove, coriander, frankincense, geranium, ginger, grapefruit, jasmine, juniper, lemon, litsea cubeba, marjoram, neroli, patchouli, petitgrain, rose absolute, sandalwood, vetiver, ylang ylang

Ormenis Flower (Chamomile Maroc)
Ormenis multicaulis

This sweet-petaled flower, which closes as the dusk sky changes into deep velvet blue, is often mistaken for another. The fragrance sighs for those who have been overlooked, those passed over by mistake, or misunderstood by others. It is no coincidence that this aroma is so often called by another name.

Those who have the gentlest of hearts and spirits are often overlooked in favor of those with more forceful spiritual natures. Yet this fragrance holds a key to the telling of who we really are, in truth with fortitude of spirit, neither meek nor mild.

It enables a person to be free enough to say, "I am also important. I too have a story to tell, and a destiny in this lifetime. I shall not always be passed over for those more flamboyant than I, those often mistaken for being stronger than I."

This fragrance reveals the true inner spirit, yet if required, will provide the camouflage sometimes needed to hide a sweet and tender-spirited heart.

Physical Healing

anti-infectious, tonic, emmenagogic, antispasmodic, sedative, calmative, antiseptic

Emotional Healing

To encourage empathy, courage, relaxation, mindfulness, attentiveness, and centering.

Aroma

balsamic, herby, sweet

Combines Well With

bay, benzoin, bergamot, cardamom, coriander, frankincense, geranium, grapefruit, lavender, lemon, lemongrass, mandarin, marjoram, orange, patchouli, petitgrain, ylang ylang, yuzu

Palmarosa
Cymbopogon martinii

*T*he fragrance of palmarosa hovers within the outer boundaries of the physical form, in the auric field and slightly beyond, energizing the human form, enabling it to extend toward the heavens.

Its strength of purpose enables it to persuade the mind to be gentle and to love the form within which it travels, knowing that all that is held in mindfulness will become a reflection of the heart. The fragrance reminds us that strength lies in direction and purpose, and that there is only one road — that of the illuminated heart. Traveling this road, we can overcome the impediments of the physical world, learn to let go, and walk with the spirit.

Palmarosa encourages us to be kind and gentle to ourselves, not overcritical or judgmental, because when we have learned to love who we are, we can love others in the same way. It tenderly creates a space, a garden, in which love can grow.

Physical Healing

antiseptic, cicatrisive, anti-depressant, stimulant, tonic

Emotional Healing

To encourage mildness, growth, loyalty, and enthusiasm.

Aroma

sweet, rosy, floral, lemony

Combines Well With

bay, benzoin, bergamot, chamomile Roman, clary sage, clove, coriander, frankincense, geranium, ginger, grapefruit, juniper, lemon, lemongrass, mandarin, orange, patchouli, petitgrain, rose absolute, rosemary, rose otto, sandalwood, ylang ylang

Patchouli
Pogostemon cablin

𝒫atchouli brings with it the sense of the sacredness of life. It is also a fragrance of action, knowing that no ideal will be reached unless we take the first steps to make it happen. At the same time, patchouli reminds us that sitting quietly under a tree is good, if there is purpose in it — the purpose of knowing and appreciating.

Sitting under a tree represents the contemplation of what we can do for ourselves and others in the way of caring. As the thought of caring for others enters our spirit, so too does the thought of caring for the tree that harbors us, and caring for all else besides. Such is the scope of patchouli's liberation from boundaries.

Physical Healing

tonic, cytophilactic, anti-infectious, antiseptic, antidepressant, calmative

Emotional Healing

To encourage farsightedness, rapport, invigoration, reasonableness, lucidity, astuteness, and stimulation.

Aroma

smoky, herbaceous, earthy

Combines Well With

bergamot, black pepper, cinnamon, clove, coriander, frankincense, geranium, ginger, grapefruit, jasmine, lemongrass, litsea cubeba, mandarin, neroli, orange, rose absolute, sandalwood, ylang ylang

Since ancient times, wherever it has been grown, patchouli has been used in incense and fragranced oils; also widely traded.

Peppermint
Mentha piperita

$\mathcal{P}$eppermint raises the spirit to fuller understanding and appreciation of the mysteries that will eventually fully unfold to us. It stimulates and soothes, uplifts and calms. Whatever is needed, this fragrance can provide it.

Those lethargic with thoughts that all is lost will be energized and come back into touch with their inner selves. Peppermint can also stimulate the dream time, using this time of physical stillness to bring information and understanding.

The fragrance will not provide a shield of comfort in restlessness, nor lull the senses. It instead increases sensitivity, awareness, and perception, bringing an alertness even in the dream state, so we can remember and take in the wisdom of other worlds.

Physical Healing

antiseptic, anti-infectious, carminative, stomachic, antispasmodic, stimulant, emmenagogic, expectorant, analgesic, digestive

Emotional Healing

To encourage regeneration, self-acceptance, concentration, vitality, and vibrancy.

Aroma

camphoraceous, minty, fresh

Combines Well With

basil, black pepper, cypress, eucalyptus, geranium, grapefruit, juniper, lavender, lemon, niaouli, pine, ravensara, rosemary, spearmint, tea tree

Peppermint (*continued*)

"Woe unto you . . . for ye pay tithe of mint and anise and cumin, and have omitted the weightier matters of the law, judgement, mercy, and faith. . . ."
— Matthew 23:23

*

According to Greek mythology, the genus *Mentha* takes its name from the nymph Minthe, who was seduced by Pluto and turned into a plant by his jealous wife, who trod her into the ground. Pluto, however, turned her into an herb, knowing Minthe would then be appreciated by people for years to come.

Petitgrain
Citrus aurantium, C. brigaradier

 $\mathcal{S}$ tability is often needed when we are at our most vulnerable, feeling fragile, and taking everything a little too personally and emotionally. It's at times such as these that we need a delicate spiritual strength, a gentle outstretched hand to guide us through the days when tears seem ever present.

The spirit of petitgrain is embodied in gentle strength, encouraging positive resolutions and outcomes at difficult times. It enables us to see ahead and to forge a link with our inner truth, helping us understand that in our personal truth comes strength.

The small twigs and little fruits from which petitgrain is made are themselves vulnerable, and in this perhaps lies the empathetic connection that petitgrain has with the human spirit. "Treading softly" also applies to our dealings with other people who might be feeling vulnerable, and are perhaps trying hard not to show it. In these circumstances, petitgrain can form a bridge across the divide that we may have created between us and them.

Physical Healing

antispasmodic, antidepressant, stimulant, tonic, calmative, anti-infectious, antiseptic, nervine

Emotional Healing

To encourage harmony, upliftment, joy, inner vision, strength, self-confidence, and expressiveness.

Aroma

warm, sharp, woody, floral

Combines Well With

basil, benzoin, bergamot, cedarwood, clary sage, clove, cypress, eucalyptus citriodora, frankincense, geranium, jasmine, juniper, lavender, lemon, mandarin, marjoram, neroli, orange, palmarosa, patchouli, rose absolute, rosemary, rose otto, sandalwood, ylang ylang, yuzu

Pimento Berry
Pimenta officinalis

*D*o not try too hard or too forcefully, advises sweet pimento, for we cannot always change what has been ordained by God. Accept gently, with compassion and thankfulness, that which has been given to us.

But pimento does not teach complacency. It encourages us to attempt to change that which we feel is having a negative effect on the collective human psyche. It helps us search within, to speak out against injustice, and be strong in the face of adversity.

Pimento softly reminds the spirit that the short time we have on earth is to be appreciated. Yet, we can both admire the beauty of the planet and enjoy our time upon it while still defending that which is right.

Physical Healing

analgesic, carminative, stimulant, tonic, antidepressant

Special Care

Not to be used during pregnancy.

*

Can cause irritation to sensitive skin.

Emotional Healing

To encourage warmth, comfort, stimulation, and energy.

Aroma

spicy, warm, balsamic

Combines Well With

bay, bergamot, camphor, cinnamon, clove, frankincense, jasmine, lavender, lemon, mandarin, orange, patchouli, petitgrain, rose absolute, ylang ylang

(use only in small amounts)

Pine
Pinus sylvestris

The pines watch humanity come and go, while they live on. Among them, below them, we inhale their powerful fragrance, which shoots through our spirit and ends in an inner explosion of understanding. In doing so, we are brought within the large embrace of nature and can inhale its presence, acceptance, and wisdom.

Pine teaches that it is love and generosity of spirit that endures — in the hearts of those we have loved and known, and in our children. Our love is that which endures, through all weathers and seasons. With this comes the knowing that we should not destroy that which is close to our hearts, for to do so is to destroy ourselves.

Physical Healing

anti-infectious, antiseptic, tonic, pectoral, expectorant, stimulant, restorative

Special Care

Can cause irritation to sensitive skin.

Emotional Healing

To encourage humility, simplicity, assurance, perseverance, mindfulness, trust, direction, and tenacity.

Aroma

crisp, clean, fresh, resinous pine

Combines Well With

bergamot, cedarwood, clary sage, cypress, eucalyptus, frankincense, grapefruit, juniper, lavender, lemon, marjoram, peppermint, ravensara, rosemary, sandalwood, tea tree, thyme linalol

Pine (*continued*)

"The glory of Lebanon shall come unto thee, the fir tree, the pine tree, and the box together, to beautify the place of my sanctuary; and I will make the place of my feet glorious."
— Isaiah 60:13

*

In parts of Poland and the Czech Republic, between Christmas and the new year, pine resin was burned throughout the long nights in the belief that the fragrant smoke would drive away any witches or other bad influences that were near.

*

In Japanese myths, the "Tree of Life" is sometimes associated with the pine. The "Fungus of Immortality" is said to grow in the shade of holy trees, of which there are several, but most usually it does so in the shade of a pine.

*

In Japanese myths, spirit lovers are sometimes said to dwell in pine trees, and live to a very old age. In classical Japanese kyogen theater, the image of a large pine tree always provides the stage backdrop.

*

In China the dragon is often associated with the pine, it being said that the pine changes into a dragon.

Rose Maroc Absolute
Rosa centifolia

The depth of this fragrance tells all who come near that this is soul perfume, or a perfume of the guardians or messengers that sometimes sally forth from the heavens to guide us and stand by us in times of need or of joy. The etheric realms associate rose absolute with the desires of the human heart. It is completing a task for which perhaps it was born — to send forth the glory of heaven, so in the smelling of the rose we can experience the subtleties of the universe. It touches and stirs the spirit, sometimes even awakening the acknowledgment of divine mysteries, and of the glory of heaven.

Physical Healing

anti-infectious, tonic, stimulant, nervine, cytophilactic

Emotional Healing

To encourage motivation, inner vitality, confidence, passion, cooperation, fulfillment, forgiveness, and a sense of freedom.

Aroma

deep, soft, hypnotic, honey-spicy rose

Combines Well With

bay, benzoin, cardamom, clove, coriander, frankincense, geranium, ginger, jasmine, lemon, mandarin, neroli, palmarosa, patchouli, sandalwood, ylang ylang

(Often adulterated during extraction with other rose species, or palmarosa or geranium.)

Rosettes are often seen on Arab, Turkish, and Israeli gravestones.

*

In India, the "Great Mother," the early goddess, was known as the "Holy Rose."

*

In ancient China, the red rose was called the "Flower of the Goddess."

Rosemary
Rosmarinus officinalis

The hills are alive with the spirit of rosemary, which spills forth its fragrance at a signal from the midday sun. Carried upon the light of the human spirit, it sends forth messages from earth to the heavens, filling the atmosphere between with its aroma. Crushed underfoot, the fragrance rises, and as it is inhaled, it enables the human spirit to receive and understand the assistance descending to us from wiser beings, and from God. Rosemary helps us to remember who we are and what our place is in the evolutionary plan. It helps us to perform tasks that may be needed on our own spiritual pathway, and to assist others along theirs if we are asked to do so.

Physical Healing

antiseptic, stimulant, analgesic, antidepressant, antispasmodic, vulnerary, carminative, emmenagogic, antitussive, decongestant

Special Care

Not to be used during pregnancy.

*

To be avoided by those with epilepsy.

Emotional Healing

To encourage energy, upliftment, confidence, clarity, concentration, stability, purification, and awareness.

Aroma

camphoraceous, woody, herbaceous, powerful

Combines Well With

basil, bergamot, black pepper, cedarwood, clary sage, cypress, eucalyptus, frankincense, geranium, grapefruit, juniper, lavender, lemon, litsea cubeba, mandarin, marjoram, naiouli, oregano, palmarosa, peppermint, pine, ravensara, tea tree, thyme linalol

In the European Tyrol, rosemary was among the fragrant plants used to fumigate and cleanse houses during the May Day festival.

Rose Otto
Rosa damascena

*T*he breath of rose otto is like the beating of angels' wings. It operates with a light far brighter even than the sun, with a frequency that cannot be measured but is still everywhere, and that we can feel if only we stop to smell the rose.

Rose otto vibrates with the energy of universal love, operating in the light of unconditional love and giving.

The rose offers itself in sacrifice for the love of the human race, and the planet. While all plants used in herbal medicine suffer in their sacrifice to help us, rose otto is the quintessential fragrance of love, the love that touches our very soul, and it is for the awakening of love in us that it offers itself.

Rose otto eases the sorrow of the soul, bringing harmony and comfort. It is gentle, yet euphoric.

Physical Healing

tonic, cicatrisive, cytophilactic, pectoral, antidepressant, calmative, hemostatic

Emotional Healing

To encourage contentment, devotion, inner vision, happiness, inner freedom, acceptance, completeness, patience, love, sensuality, and purity.

Aroma

flowery, rosy, lemony, fresh

Combines Well With

amber, benzoin, bergamot, chamomile Roman, geranium, jasmine, lemon, mandarin, neroli, petitgrain, sandalwood, ylang ylang

Rose Otto (*continued*)

The Virgin Mary has been called the "Rose," "Holy Rose," the "Rose Garden," the "Queen of the Most Holy Rose Garden," "Mystic Rose," "Rose Garland," and "Rose Bush."

*

In ancient Greece, the rose was symbolic of the goddess Aphrodite. In Roman times it was said the rose sprung from the blood of the god Adonis, while others still maintained it sprung from the blood of the goddess Venus, the Roman name for Aphrodite.

*

In ancient Greece and Italy, graves were planted with rosebushes and strewn with rose petals.

*

In medieval Europe, religious rites for the dead were often carried out in rose gardens or within the "rose hedge."

Sage
Salvia officinalis

*S*acred sage cleanses and purifies the spirit. The spirit of the different sages, for there are many, holds the wisdom of the spheres within its fragrance, while summoning the powers that heal and protect.

Sage is a protective spirit for those who are not afraid of the spiritual forces or of the force of unseen beings. The might of the heavens summoned by the sage is wisdom and power, which help us to stand fast in times of adversity.

Sage's purpose is all these things for the human. Also, it helps us to integrate a spirit that has the majesty of the heavens behind it, to call forth God and the celestial warriors to defend, protect, and heal the human spirit and Mother Earth.

Physical Healing

antiseptic, antispasmodic, diuretic, emmenagogic, tonic

Special Care

Must not be used during pregnancy.

*

Must not be used by those with epilepsy.

Emotional Healing

To encourage strength, courage, perseverance, grounding, and to offer protection.

Aroma

warm, herby, spicy, camphoraceous

Combines Well With

basil, cedarwood, chamomile maroc, cypress, hyssop, lavender, lemon, myrtle, orange, peppermint, petitgrain, pine, rosemary, thyme, yarrow

(Rarely used in aromatherapy — best used in vaporizing/diffuser methods.)

Sage (*continued*)

There are many varieties of sage growing around the world, some of which are said to have spiritual powers and are an important component of religious ceremony. The ancient Romans called sage *herba sacra*, or the sacred herb, and would have been referring to the species with the Latin name *Salvia officinalis*. Sage is today most commonly used for spiritual purposes by the Native American nations, who use the word *sage* for several species of plant that would more properly fall into the botanical group *Compositae*.

*

In Mexico the Mazatec people use *Salvia divinorum* for divination. The North American Paiutes use *Artemisia dracynculoides* in the costume of the medicine man and in various spiritual practices and rituals, including the sun dance celebration. *Artemisia tridentata* is incorporated in the costume of Washoe medicine men, and is also used in the making of the moccasins used during the sun dances. It is burned at the start of all spiritual ceremonies, and is also an essential part of the ritual bathing ceremony.

Sandalwood
Santalum album

A fragrance that stretches out to the universe, into the hallowed space between heaven and earth, to contact the divine presence. Sandalwood brings our wisdom into a meditative state, quieting us so we can hear and rejoice in the choral singing of the universal soul. It brings us into the great cosmic prayer, the infinite meditation.

Sandalwood helps humanity to have strength of conviction when standing against adversity, as it joins all aspects of being. It rejoices in the physical aspects of mankind, while always being aware of the spiritual self.

Physical Healing

antiseptic, antidepressant, diuretic, tonic, calmative, anti-infectious, decongestant

Emotional Healing

To encourage warmth, sensitivity, serenity, harmony, peace, wisdom, insightfulness, and unity.

Aroma

warm, balsamic, rich, woody

Combines Well With

benzoin, black pepper, chamomile Roman, clary sage, clove, fennel, frankincense, geranium, grapefruit, jasmine, lavender, lemon, mandarin, myrrh, neroli, orange, palmarosa, patchouli, petitgrain, rose absolute, rose otto, ylang ylang

Sandalwood (*continued*)

The oldest Vedic scripture, the fifth-century BCE *Nirukta*, mentions sandalwood, which has continued to be one of the most important fragrances used in Indian religious practice. The early written records show sandalwood was traded from earliest times.

*

Sandalwood has been widely used in embalming. In Ceylon, princes were embalmed from the ninth century onward.

*

Other species produce an oil that is similar in smell only (not in terms of therapeutic values) — the African *Osyris tenuifolia* plant, the Australian *Antalum spicatum*, and the West Indian *Amyris balsamifera*.

Spikenard
Nardostachys jatamansi

*F*or the sweet depths of devotion. In preparation for the departure of the spirit to the heavens, spikenard allows us to release our fears of the unknown, to have the courage to step forward. Spikenard helps to reconcile all that has happened to us in this lifetime upon the earth, and to make peace with those who have hurt us. It is a fragrance of forgiveness offered with love, as well as a fragrance that carries with it the bonds of human existence, the chains that bind us to the emotions that we may be fearful of letting go. Its purpose is to release the past from the shackles of our own making, those that relentlessly bind us to repeating actions that affect the freedom of the spirit.

Physical Healing

antiseptic, calmative, sedative, anti-infectious

Emotional Healing

To encourage forgiveness, fearlessness, calm, centering, balance, and resolution.

Aroma

heavy, warm, peaty, musty

Combines Well With

clary sage, clove, cypress, frankincense, geranium, juniper, lavender, lemon, myrrh, neroli, palmarosa, patchouli, pine, rose absolute, vetiver

Known in ancient times as "nard."

*

"Then took Mary a pound of ointment of spikenard, very costly, and anointed the feet of Jesus."   — John 12:3

Storax (Styrax)
Liquidambar orientalis

In meditation and prayer, the divine purpose of souls has a voice through this fragrance. It unlocks doors leading to unknown corridors in the furthermost reaches of the mind, where there are windows to the souls of light.

This ancient and mystical fragrance brings us back to the source of creation, to the time when all was one, helping us to understand the paths taken by the saints and martyrs who sacrificed all for the love of God.

Answers come in their own time, but storax softly opens and prepares each heart for that knowing.

Physical Healing

antiseptic, antitussive, expectorant, nervine

Aroma

sweet, resinous, balsamic, vanilla-like

Special Care

Not to be used during pregnancy.

*

Can cause irritation to sensitive skin.

Emotional Healing

To encourage soothing, harmony, benevolence, compassion, and unity.

Combines Well With

bay, cardamom, carnation, cinnamon, clove, geranium, ginger, helichrysum, hyacinth, jasmine, lavender, lemon, nutmeg, orange, rose absolute, ylang ylang

Another species with a very similar aroma, *Styrax officinalis* is a big bushy shrub with white flowers and is commonly thought to be the "stacte" of the holy incense, in Exodus 30:34.

*

The name "styrax" is sometimes given to *Liquidambar orientalis* — storax.

Thyme (Red and Chemotype Linalol)
Thymus vulgaris

There is fire within the soul of thyme, the fire to summon the most mighty angels to our assistance — the force within the compassion, the forgiveness in might, the enlightenment of the mind and spirit, the revealing of truth. In the power and might of the heavens, where pretense does not exist, we cannot hide — least of all from ourselves.

This fragrance joins with our guardians in assisting us in having strength and love for ourselves during times of reconciliation, when we strive to acknowledge the shadows and disrobe the outer shell of protection — the disguise that we may find difficult even to acknowledge.

Physical Healing

analgesic, expectorant, antiseptic, anti-infectious, emmenagogic

Special Care

Not to be used during pregnancy.

*

Can cause irritation to sensitive skin.

Emotional Healing

To encourage balance, tolerance, courage, supportiveness, alertness, and warmth.

Aroma

sharp, woody, herbaceous
(*The species known as thyme linalol is gentler and has a softer, more woody, herbaceous aroma.*)

Combines Well With

birch, clary sage, cypress, eucalyptus, frankincense, geranium, ginger, grapefruit, hyssop, lemon, mandarin, myrtle, orange, ormenis flower, palmarosa, pimento berry, pine, rosemary

Tuberose (Absolute)
Polianthes tuberosa

𝒯uberose embodies forgiveness and the rediscovering of self love when the self is lost and the spirit low. When the ego has received many life blows, and is depressed and unable to connect with the higher realms, tuberose assists in that reconnection. This is a perfume for when finding oneself in a world in which it is easy to be without hope. When all seems lost, it brings the ego into the spirit, in an event that brings balance and harmony.

It helps in transporting the spirit to places unknown, where it can dwell for a brief moment, finding comfort and knowing.

Tuberose is for the finding of truth in truths long forgotten, for bringing hopes and dreams and prayers to their rightful place, and in so doing, it integrates the highest elements of the ego within spiritual wonderment.

Physical Healing

antidepressant, calmative, nervine, sedative

Emotional Healing

To encourage motivation, enthusiasm, encouragement, sensuality, sensitivity, expressiveness, and frankness.

Aroma

Sweet, heavy, spicy, floral

Combines Well With

balsam de Peru, benzoin, bergamot, hyacinth, jasmine, mandarin, narcissus, orange, ormenis flower, rose absolute, sandalwood

In India, Malaysia, and other Asian countries, the flowers are made into garlands and placed around the necks of religious sculptures, such as Krishna, Shiva, and Buddha, and also given as offerings at home shrines.

*

In Egypt, garlands are made during religious festivals.

Vetiver
Vetiveria zizanioides

Sometimes deep secrets of the soul are hidden in the heart, buried so deep as not to disturb the waking dream of who we think we are. Vetiver can awaken those secrets, which often involve the realization that we are not alone in the universe. This awakening can be unsteadying, even unbalancing, but vetiver holds us steadfast. Vetiver stops the swirling of the mind, the turmoil of unanswerable questions.

In many ways, vetiver helps us to remain calm when unsettling events and adversity affect the spiritual self.

Gently, and without disturbing the creative forces, vetiver steadies and calms any inner disquiet, and in that calmness may come the answers we seek.

Physical Healing

antiseptic, tonic, emmenagogic, antispasmodic, nervine

Emotional Healing

To encourage growth, integrity, wisdom, strength, honor, protection, self-esteem, and grounding.

Aroma

soft, earthy, musty

Combines Well With

bergamot, black pepper, clary sage, coriander, eucalyptus citriodora, geranium, ginger, grapefruit, jasmine, lavender, lemon, lemongrass, litsea cubeba, mandarin, melissa, orange, rose absolute, sandalwood, ylang ylang, yuzu

Violet Leaf (Absolute)
Viola odorata

*V*iolet is for timidity of the spirit. There are those who have within them deep knowing, who silently marvel at the wonder of life, who yet are shy. They may fear venturing forth into worlds unknown, or fear the afterlife. They may be unable to voice the troubles of their heart and soul. There are those too who are unable to pray out loud, and instead silently offer a prayer from their heart, although sometimes wondering if it will be heard. Some are too timid to step into the light and feel its strength-giving warmth, that which gives courage to speak and be heard. And there are those too timid to accept the love offered by all realms. For all these shy, timid spirits, violet offers understanding and empathy, and a way into the great open void of love.

Physical Healing

analgesic, antirheumatic, decongestant, diuretic, soporific

Emotional Healing

To encourage security, courage, confidence, centering, gentleness, and upliftment.

Aroma

forceful greenish with slight floral edge

Combines Well With

basil, bay, cinnamon,clary sage, clove, geranium, grapefruit, hyacinth, jasmine, lavender, lemon, rose absolute, sandalwood, tangerine, tuberose

(use only small amounts in blends)

Yarrow
Achillea millefolium

*T*his fragrance has long been an energetic messenger of the heavens, since it was first planted by the Creator. It delicately balances the flow between the yin and yang energies received from the sun, the moon, and the stars. Once the balance and harmonization of yin and yang energy within a person has been completed, the fragrance acts as a conduit for the opening of intuitive perception and the acceptance of the hidden faculties of the mind. Although it at all times remains firmly attached to the earth plane, it intercepts and assists in the delivery of messages and prophecies from other planes of existence.

It is fragrance for dreaming, for visionary experiences, for traveling on the energy of the universe, while being protected and nurtured.

Physical Healing

anti-inflammatory, antiseptic, carminative, tonic, antispasmodic

Special Care

Can cause irritation to sensitive skin.

Emotional Healing

To encourage harmony, equilibrium, intuition, centering, dreams, and visions.

Aroma

herby green with a slightly spicy camphoraceous note

Combines Well With

bergamot, birch, black pepper, chamomile Roman, clary sage, cypress, eucalyptus, fennel, frankincense, geranium, ginger, helichrysum, lavender, lemon, marjoram, myrtle, peppermint, pine, rosemary, sage

Yarrow (*continued*)

A sacred plant to the Native American nations and the Chinese, among others.

*

The long, woodlike dried stems of the yarrow plant continue to be used as the most traditionally correct tool for casting the *I Ching,* for prophecy.

Ylang Ylang
Cananga odorata

*Y*lang ylang is the tenderhearted one whose hanging petals dance in the wind, as if through flexibility it protects its tender heart from destruction. It shields and guides the passion of love and true emotion, while allowing a tender awakening of that sensual part of our being and spirit that can embrace all things. It will open our hearts to the pleasures that God has given to us as we walk our mortal path, and help us to understand that even heaven and the angelic realms enjoy the passion of a spiritual being. It may soften the hard-hearted and allow those who use judgment against others to feel the soft seduction of heaven. Ylang ylang is for those who have a yearning for completion.

Physical Healing

sedative, antiseptic, aphrodisiac, nervine, antidepressant, calmative

Emotional Healing

To encourage self-confidence, warmth, awakening, sensuality, upliftment, calm, joy, and enthusiasm.

Aroma

sweet, intense, balsamic, floral

Combines Well With

bergamot, chamomile Roman, clary sage, clove, eucalyptus citriodora, ginger, grapefruit jasmine, lemon, litsea cubeba, mandarin, orange, palmarosa, patchouli, petitgrain, rose absolute, sandalwood, vetiver, yuzu

Yuzu
Citrus junos

*Y*uzu is purifying, strong, and clearly focused. If we are feeling spiritually unsettled, yuzu gives us the spiritual purification and strength we need to move forward, and the focus we require as we take in new thoughts and feelings. It also has within it the facility of discipline, which we require so as not to allow our thoughts to stray or allow oursleves to become unsettled and distracted by others.

Stillness and focus are the reference points that make invisible the many distractions that tempt us from the spiritual peace. This yuzu offers — sweetly, kindly, and with a resolution that can withstand all storms — a benignly confident smile upon its face.

Physical Healing

tonic, stimulant, anti-infectious, diuretic, calmative, antiseptic, analgesic

Special Care

Avoid using on the skin if exposed to sunlight or ultraviolet rays.

Emotional Healing

To encourage focus, concentration, strength, courage, and centering.

Aroma

a unique blend of fresh citrus

Combines Well With

basil, bergamot, black pepper, cardamom, cedarwood, clary sage, coriander, cypress, ginger, jasmine, lavender, marjoram, palmarosa, pine, ravensara, rose absolute, rosemary, sandalwood, ylang ylang

It's used in religious ceremonies by some Shinto priests for purification before prayer.

GLOSSARY OF THERAPEUTIC PROPERTIES
(as itemized in the section Physical Healing)

Analgesic: Reduces pain sensation

Antibiotic/antibacterial: Prevents bacterial growth

Antifungal: Prevents fungal growth

Anti-infectious: Prevents uptake of infection

Antiparasitic: Acts against insect parasites

Antiseptic: Destroys microbes and prevents their development

Antispasmodic: Prevents or relieves spasms, convulsions, and contractions

Antisudorific: Prevents sweating

Antitussive: Relieves coughs

Antiviral: Prevents viral growth

Balsamic: Soothing to sore throats, coughs, etc.

Calmative: Sedative, calming agent

Carminative: Relieves flatulence, easing abdominal pain and bloating

Cholagogic: Promotes the evacuation of bile from gall bladder and ducts

Cicatrisive: Promotes the formation of scar tissue, thus healing

Cytophilactic: Promotes cell turnover, thus healing

Depurative: Cleanser, detoxifier; purifies blood and internal organs

Diuretic: Promotes the removal of excess water from the body by urine

Emmenagogic: Induces or regularizes menstruation

Emollient: Soothes and softens skin

Expectorant: Promotes removal of mucus from the body

Febrifuge: An antifebrile agent (antifever)

Galactagogic: Induces the flow of milk

Hemostatic: Stops bleeding

Hepatic: Acts on the liver

Immunostimulant: Stimulates the action of the immune system

Nervine: Acts on nerves; relieves nervous disorders

Pectoral: Beneficial for diseases or conditions of the chest and respiratory system

Rubefacient: A counterirritant, producing redness of the skin

Sedative: Reduces mental excitement or physical activity

Soporific: Induces, or tends to induce, sleep

Stimulant: Increases overall function of the body

Stomachic: Good for the stomach; gastric tonic, digestive aid

Tonic: Invigorates, refreshes, and restores body functions

Vermifuge: Expels intestinal worms

Vulnerary: Heals wounds and sores by external application

Chapter 12

The Aromatic Traditions

Humanity will be saved through the flower.
— Huvenol, Mayan elder,
quoting a Mayan prophecy

FRAGRANCE HAS PLAYED A VERY IMPORTANT PART in the spiritual traditions of the world, with no other material substance being so universally employed in spiritual practice. We know fragrance can affect both body and mind, but it can also affect spiritual perceptions, and it is this aspect, I believe, above any of the many philosophical/metaphorical/practical aspects, that ultimately explains its widespread use.

From a philosophical point of view, aroma is both physical and ethereal, linking the realms of the known and unknown. Fragrance is also transformational — with resin, for example, being changed from light, odorless rock into fragrant smoke, rising to heaven. The delightful nature of fragrance reminds people of the good things in life and of all they have to be grateful for, and with it, they give thanks. By a simple analogy, death, decay, and bad smells were historically equated with evil and good smells equated with wellness, immortality, and the spiritual realms. Burning fragrant material sent a "smoke signal" to the gods, letting them know people were thinking of them and seeking their help. The medicinal qualities of many fragrant materials were used, in ancient Mesopotamia for example, in inhalations, medicated baths, and poultices, and their beneficent properties must have been thought a blessing from the gods.

There are, then, many reasons why fragrance might have been considered the means by which to show appreciation to the deity. It is also the case that fragrance affects the mind and spirit, and no doubt the people who used fragrance on a regular basis knew this too, as do those who continue to use it for that purpose today.

THE GODDESS OF THE SACRED TREES

*Lady of breath, fragrant woman of air, whose words are hot and sweet in
his nostrils. . . . She is eternity, essence, window onto forever.*

— *The Egyptian Book of the Dead*

The earliest known building with a specifically ritual purpose, a place of communal worship, is nine thousand years old. It's at Novali Cori, on the Turkey-Syria border. The people here, like all others known to archaeologists from this time, worshipped a goddess, here associated with a tortoise. Goddess worship was known throughout Europe, the Middle East, India, Pakistan, and northern Africa, from possibly as early as 30,000 BCE. Male gods began to appear only around 6000 BCE, and started out as sons of the goddesses, then became their consorts, eventually taking over the main spiritual role. However, it was a long process, which involved the prophets of the Old Testament fighting "the queen of heaven" and her "idolaters," and the ancient Greeks, who as late as 500 BCE were still arguing over who should have supremacy — the male (Zeus) or the female (Athene). Male gods eventually won out.

The battle against the worship of females is told in the Old Testament. For example, in Jeremiah 44:17, the people of Pathros told the prophet

> "we will not hearken unto thee: But we will certainly do whatsoever thing goeth forth out of our own mouths, to burn incense unto the queen of heaven, and to pour out drink offerings unto her, as we have done, we, and our fathers, our kings, and our princes, in the cities of Judah, and in the streets of Jerusalem: for then had we plenty of victuals, and were well, and saw no evil."

The Canaanites worshipped a goddess called Astarte, and put plaques with images ("graven images") of her on the backs of their doors so when the agents of the Israelite kings burst into the houses to check on their religious practices, as the doors were thrown open, the images would be hidden between the door and the walls. The Canaanites also worshipped the goddess as a tree, such as pine, juniper, and cypress, and where these were not available, they substituted *asherah*, wooden poles made of tree trunks that were placed in the ground.

Incense burning was a central feature of goddess worship, in predynastic and later Egypt, in Sumeria, and throughout the Middle East. As time passed and the authority of the goddesses became supplanted by that of male gods, the priestesses who had served the goddesses were replaced by male priests. Censers have been found in the graves of many women, humble as well as noble, and it's thought that many ordinary women took on the role of priestess within their local area. As the official power and authority of women in spiritual matters dwindled, their area of influence became confined to that of oracle-giving. This involved going into trance — often induced by inhaling the smoke of burning incense and other fragrant material — and apparently speaking in the voices of the gods or goddesses.

The most famous oracle was at Delphi in Greece, from whom national leaders sought advice long after the male element had taken over official religions. The oracle was known as Pythia, "the Pythoness," or snake priestess. The fragrant material favored at Delphi was bay, which was burned to produce a profusion of smoke. It's also been suggested that the roof of the central building at Delphi was made of branches of bay trees, and that the oracle ate the leaves. By the late Greek period, goddesses had more or less been softened and made sensual rather than all-powerful. Many continued to be associated with fragrance, such as Circe, Demeter, and Aphrodite, also known as Venus.

ANCIENT EGYPT

> It was . . . in their grand religious processions that they made the most luxurious display of perfumes. In one of those described as having taken place under one of the Ptolemies, marched 120 children, bearing incense, myrrh, and saffron in golden basins, followed by a number of camels, some carrying three hundred pounds weight of frankincense, and others a similar quantity of crocus, cassia, cinnamon, orris, and other precious ointments.
> — Eugene Rimmel, *The Book of Perfumes*

The ancient Egyptians didn't question whether there was a life after death. They were so convinced, they spent half their lives preparing for it. Royalty and people of standing or wealth built tombs for themselves — which would be packed with all manner of possessions needed in the afterlife, as the body itself would be packed with aromatic materials during mummification to prevent decay.

The Egyptian civilization grew up along the banks of the Nile River, starting around 4000 BCE, with the first walled cities appearing around 3300 BCE, the unification of the "upper" and "lower" valley kingdoms occurring in 3100 BCE, and the construction of the first stepped pyramid beginning around 2650 BCE Egypt continued as an important cultural center for another twenty-six hundred years, until the defeat of Cleopatra in 30 BCE by the Roman leader Octavian-Augustus. Because there was such long continuity in the priestly tradition that recorded knowledge about plants, and because this evidence remains either in papyrus or stone, we can be very sure that fragrance in all its forms was lavishly used throughout the millennia.

The existence of the myrrh tree was explained as it being a tear of the god Horus, as other incense trees grew where the tears of the gods Shu and Tefnet fell. The gods were offered incense in return, usually in the form of little round pastilles, or balls, that the priest fed into the long censer, balanced carefully on one hand.

The sun-god Ra was offered some form of resin at dawn, myrrh at midday, and kyphi at sunset. This last incense was admired by many famous Greeks, including Galen, and has been passed down to us in the form of several recipes. Plutarch said it could heal the soul. There were at least sixteen ingredients, possibly including wine, honey, raisins, myrrh, cardamom, juniper, mint, cypress, spikenard, cassia, and cinnamon. Within the temple complexes there were special areas for preparing incense for ritual use, and as this was carried out, priests would read aloud from sacred texts. A visual record of the making of kyphi can still be seen on the walls of the Temple of Horus at Edfu.

In the late 1960s, at Saqqara, Dominique Mallet and other archaeologists excavated the tomb of Ptah Du-Auu, a nobleman and high priest. Most items had been removed by grave robbers, but they did find two used censers and some pots, one of which had "B'rth Respeth incense" written on the side in ink, and inside, about half a pound of resinous material, which apparently included benzoin, sandalwood, myrrh, frankincense, and juniper, along with lotus oil, fragrant rush, sweet gum bark, and gum mastic.

In many temples, priests and priestesses would burn fragrant woods and resins throughout the day, but as can be seen from the beautiful wall friezes left for us to enjoy, on important state occasions the king himself would lead the ritual, holding a censer in one hand and a spouted vase in the other. This vase may have contained wine, or possibly the perfumed oil that was poured on the altar or put on statues of the gods.

The ancient Egyptians needed oils to keep their skin supple in the searing dry heat, and these were perfumed in various ways: by steeping the petals or other fragrant material in oil or fats; by putting the material in hot oils and straining; by squeezing the essence out of plants using a press; or by putting the plant in fabric that was then twisted very tight using special equipment.

Embalming involved much anointing of the body and filling body cavities with copious amounts of fragrant material and resins such as cassia, cedarwood, and myrrh. Frankincense was reserved for use on the head. Vases of fragrant oils were placed with the mummy, who, it was thought, would surely need them when the transition to the other world was complete. When buried, the body was first anointed and perfumed, and a crown of flowers was placed on the head. A prayer was then said, invoking the god Horus to favor the dead with his perfume and acceptance.

The Egyptians traded extensively to acquire the aromatics they required in both their spiritual and secular lives. Temples and homes were both fragranced, sometimes with a censer with a perforated cover. As well as the fragrant materials already mentioned, which are used today in the form of essential oils, spikenard, galbanum, and at a later date rose were known to have been used.

As Egypt declined in power and importance, the accumulated knowledge of plants transferred to the many excellent schools of medicine and learning that emerged from the third century BCE onward. The most famous of these was located at the busy northern port of Alexandria, which became the center of alchemical research that aimed to sublimate matter and give body to that which is spiritual. Alchemists sought to capture the essential spark of divinity in plant and mineral matter. As part of this quest, essential oils were distilled or "transformed" from raw plant material, giving rise to the enduring idea that essential oils have *quintus essentialis*, or "life force."

In *The Gold Making of Cleopatra* (not the queen), an Alexandrian text of the first century CE, there is the first illustration of a distillation unit, the invention of which is ascribed to "Maria the Jewess." Alongside are two other images: one is a serpent holding its tail in its mouth and the inscription "All is one"; the other is a circular disk within which are the words "It is toward oneness that all phenomena tend." Pliny, the first-century Roman writer, visited the perfume factories of Alexandria, noting twenty-eight different varieties, and described how the workers had to remove their clothing before leaving in the evening because the costly perfume materials may have adhered to them. Fragrance was precious indeed.

MESOPOTAMIA

> I poured out a libation on the peak of the mountain
> Seven and yet seven kettles I set up
> Under them I heaped up sweet cane, cedar, myrtle,
> The gods smelled the savor,
> The gods smelled the sweet savor
> The gods gathered like flies over the sacrificer.
> — Epic of Gilgamesh, 2000 BCE

Mesopotamia is the name given to the area between the two great rivers Euphrates and Tigris, which run southeast from the mountains of Turkey, through Syria and Iraq, to the Persian Gulf. Around 3500 BCE the first city-states appeared in the south, which came to be known as Sumeria. Ur, Uruk, and Lagash grew prosperous on an agricultural economy, greatly aided by vast irrigation schemes. The temples dominated the city physically. At Ur, for example, the vast ziggurat rose to the heavens by three steps, the lowest of these being forty-five feet high. Ritual was at the center of social activity. The temple owned much of the land, and controlled most foreign trade, which went west to Egypt and east to the Indus Valley. The need to keep records of the crop surplus, and the import and export of goods, gave impetus to the invention of writing. These "cuneiform" records make it possible to accurately ascertain events of the past. One tablet, for example, says that five thousand years ago people were placing orders for "oils of cypress, myrrh, and cedar to be obtained from abroad."

As time went on, city-states such as Kish, Nippur, and Babylon, farther northwest upriver, became more prominent. This more northern region is generally known as Babylonia. The city of Babylon became an important center of trade, as did the northerly rain-fed Nineveh, their economic and political importance continuing into Assyrian times. Much of the trading was in various spices, which were used for ritual, cleansing, medicine, perfuming, and cooking.

The Mesopotamians liked to take their rituals as high as possible, to a mountaintop, or very high clay-brick construction, where huge amounts of incense would be burned to attract the gods and goddesses. The fragrant materials available included juniper, myrtle, calamus, pine, and fir resins, as well as cedar, cypress, myrrh and, certainly by the later period, around 600 BCE, frankincense and sandalwood. Many other fragrant plants may have been used, as evidenced by the existence of a text on herbs dated to 2200 BCE, which lists 250 species and gives recipes for perfumes and ointments.

Anointing had great significance in several contexts. Oil was rubbed onto statues of deities and on stones meant to represent ancestors; poured on the head of a girl as a sign she was chosen to be married, or on the head of a vassal king; and used to confirm a contract or oath. How much of this anointing oil was fragranced is difficult to tell, but historians do know that Babylon was renowned for its scents, which were traded far and wide. Liquid essences were stored in alabaster or glass bottles, while ointments were kept in boxes made of porcelain or chalcedony.

In Babylonian religious literature the mother-goddess Ishtar has a son, Tammuz, who "dies" each year, to be reborn — in symbolism for the "death" of nature and its rebirth in spring. In *The Descent of Ishtar to the Underworld*, it says of Tammuz: "Wash him with clean water, anoint him with perfumed oil, dress him in a red cloth. . . ." Commenting on this in *The Golden Bough*, J. G. Frazer states that religious songs or chants were made over an effigy of the dead god "while the fumes of incense rose into the air, as if to stir his dormant senses by their pungent fragrance and wake him from the sleep of death."

The cuneiform tablets frequently mention incense as well as the censers that distributed the aroma around both temples and homes. Incense seems to have been used in some quantity, with a King Nabonnedos, for example, apparently "filling the temple with the odor of incense." Often censers would be mentioned along with incantations that were supposed to drive out evil spirits. Houses where there was sickness were fumigated with incense and torches of burning fragrant material to exorcise negative influences.

In Mesopotamia, plants were seen as the source of deity and immortality, with kings offering incense to the "Sacred Tree," and the epic hero Gilgamesh going in search of "the herb of immortality." Being on the crossroads between the East and the West, the people had access to a variety of fragrant material, which was used in protective amulets, lotions, compresses, inhalation, medicinal baths, and massage oils. The fragrance molecules could have been extracted by seeping the raw material in oil or fat, although pots found at Tepe Gawra, near Nineveh, also suggest that some form of distillation method was in use.

THE HEBREW TRADITION AND THE KABBALAH

> *As each commandment [of the Ten Commandments] was spoken by the*
> *Holy One, Blessed be He, the world filled with fragrance.*
> — Shabbat 88b, Rabbi Yehoshua ben-Levi

The first Jewish patriarch was Abraham, who lived in Mesopotamia around 1700 BCE. As we read in Genesis 12:1, the Lord told Abraham, "Get thee out of thy country . . . unto a land that I will show thee: And I will make of thee a great nation. . . ." Abraham duly went with his wife, Sarah, and nephew, Lot, to Canaan, settling away from the already cultivated lands of the farming Canaanites, by the "oak of Moreh." In time, to prevent his flocks from overgrazing the land, Abraham went to the hills of Hebron and Lot went to Sodom, on the plain of Jordan. Years later, because of a famine in Canaan, Abraham's descendants went to Egypt, where they were enslaved for centuries, before being led out of captivity by Moses. They returned to Canaan, where people were already living in the fertile valleys, and went to the uninhabited forested hills. This was the land flowing "with milk and honey" — the milk came from the goats, and the honey from the bees that fed on the many fragrant wildflowers growing among the wild undergrowth. The hills were cleared, terraced, and planted with olive, fig, and pomegranate trees, as well as vineyards.

In Exodus 30, Moses was instructed by God to make both a holy incense and a sacred anointing oil. The practice of offering incense twice daily started with Aaron, during the long flight through the wilderness from Egypt, and continued at the Temple in Jerusalem. In the Hebrew holy scriptures (according to the Masoretic text), the ingredients are given as "sweet spices, stacte, and onycha, and galbanum; sweet spices with pure frankincense." The Temple Institute in Jerusalem told me that the complete list was stacte, onycha, galbanum, frankincense, myrrh, cassia, spikenard, saffron, costus, aromatic bark, and cinnamon. Some versions of the Christian Bible, along with the Hebrew, add "seasoned with salt, pure and holy." The "salt" was probably saltpeter, a binding agent.

There is an ongoing and complex debate about the names given to plants and plant materials in the Bible. The cinnamon we know, *Cinnamomum verum* (formerly *Cinnamomum zeylanicum*), only grew in the East, although it is documented that the Phoenicians and Arabs were trading it perhaps as early as 500 BCE, and maybe even earlier. It's also possible that the "cinnamon" of ancient texts has been translated incorrectly, and that it refers to the bark of an Ethiopian tree, called *Amyris kataf*. Similar issues of definition surround cassia, stacte, onycha, and hyssop, among others. Even considering more local plants can be problematic. Stacte might have been, for example, *Styrax officinale*, *Liquidambar orientalis*, *Pistacia lentiscus*, or the sweetly fragrant resin that used to exude spontaneously from *Amyris kataf*, the bark of which, in other opinions, is the biblical "cinnamon." You can see how complicated it gets!

What is certain is that the hillsides of ancient Israel abounded with fragrant flowers, herbs, and shrubs; that resins exuded from many species of trees; and that fragrance was an important part of ancient Hebrew life. The medicinal properties of these fragrant materials were at least partly understood, and their purification and cleansing properties much appreciated. Fragrant incense accompanied offerings and prayers to God, while the fragrant holy oil — made of myrrh, cinnamon, calamus, and cassia diluted in olive oil — was used to anoint the tabernacle, the ark, the table, the candlestick, the altar of incense, and the altar of burned offering, along with all their associated cups and containers.

> *Aaron shall burn fragrant incense; every morning when he tends the*
> *lamps he shall burn the incense, and when he lights the lamps between*
> *dusk and dark, he shall burn the incense; so there shall be a perpetual*
> *burning of incense before the Lord of all your generations.*
>
> — Exodus 30:7–8

When Moses was instructed to make both the holy incense and oil, it was advised that he should make them, depending on the text one reads, either "after the art of the apothecary" or "after the art of the perfumer." At this time, of course, they were in a sense one and the same thing, as perfumes — fragrance materials — were central components in the apothecary's, that is, druggist's or pharmacist's, *materia medica*.

> *And Hezekiah hearkened unto them, and shewed them all the house of*
> *his precious things, the silver, and the gold, and the spices, and the pre-*
> *cious ointment . . .*
>
> — Isaiah 39:2 and 2 Kings 20:13

The ancient Hebrews used aromatics as part of personal hygiene and cleansing practices, as body perfumes and clothes fragrancers, as pest-deterrent fumigations, as fragrancers of bedding and linen, and as seasoning for food and wine. They were used for anointing the heads of guests in welcoming them to the house and in funerary rites. Fragrance was precious but also an essential part of daily life.

The mystical aspect of Judaism is, in part, contained in the tradition known as Kabbalah. These teachings aim to explore and explain, in both biblical and metaphysical terms, the relationship between God, the universe, and mankind. Being very much an oral tradition, Kabbalah has changed over the years and has had different perspectives on the nature of things. In one medieval text, Eliphas Levi presented the following incense formulas, which he related to colors:

ELIPHAS LEVI'S INCENSE FORMULAS

COLOR	INCENSE COMPOSED OF:
Red	balm, ambergris, grains of paradise, saffron
Green	benzoin, mace, storax
Blue	roses, violets
Purple	saffron, cinnamon, red sanders
White	camphor, amber, aloes, white sandal, cucumber seeds

There has always been a strong connection in the Jewish tradition between fragrance and light, since Aaron was instructed to light the lamps at the same time as burn the incense on the altar. The lamps are the seven-part candlestick known as the menorah, which has been the symbol of Israel for three thousand years, and the shape of which is modeled after a plant. There are so many highly fragrant plants growing in Israel that have the shape of the menorah, it's difficult to say which exact species it was fashioned after, and the generic term *moriah* is applied to them all. *Salvia dominica* and *Salvia palaestina* are likely candidates, and are both varieties of sage. On the evening of the Sabbath, Jews remember the lamps and incense of the Temple in Jerusalem, when blessings are made over the *havdallah* candle and spice box. Different spices are used, but myrtle has been called "the quintessential fragrant plant of Israel" and is often preferred, when available. Indeed, the spice box is called *hadass*, which means "myrtle," by many Ashkenazic and Sephardic Jews.

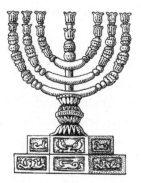

The menorah:
the seven-branched candlestick

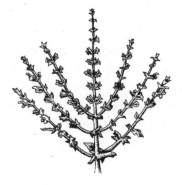

A moriah plant

THE CHRISTIAN TRADITION

> . . . *Mary Magdalene, and Mary the mother of James, and Salome, had*
> *bought sweet spices, that they might come and anoint him.*
>
> — Mark 16:1

From his birth to his death, Jesus knew about fragrance. At his birth in Bethlehem, two of the three wise men brought the gifts of frankincense and myrrh. After his crucifixion and placing in the sepulchre, the two Marys and Salome came to anoint him with "sweet spices," as was the custom for the dear departed at the time.

> *But I have all, and abound: I am full, having received of Epaphroditus the things which were sent from you, an odour of a sweet smell, a sacrifice acceptable, well pleasing to God.*
>
> — Philippians 4:18

The word *savor* in the Bible is often interchangeable with the word *fragrance*, depending on which version you read. In biblical times, savor was used to describe the smell of sacrifice, which in the tabernacle was of both meat and incense, there being two altars for these purposes — one of brass and the other gold. This practice of making dual sacrifice can make reading Bible references confusing, as it's difficult to know whether "sweet savor," which is pleasing to God, means the aroma of the burning meat or of the burning incense, or both.

The word *savor* was also used to indicate "sacrifice," in its broadest sense, as when St. Paul spoke to the Ephesians: "And walk in love, as Christ also hath loved us, and hath given himself for us an offering and a sacrifice to God for a sweet-smelling savor." To the Corinthians, he said: "For we are unto God a sweet savor of Christ...." *Savor* was so well understood to mean sacrifice it was used metaphorically, so that *not* to have savor, according to *The Illustrated Bible Dictionary*, indicated insipidity or foolishness and lack of strength. It states, "Something is missing from God's people or the worship of God when there is no 'savor.'"

> *Is any sick among you? Let him call for the elders of the church; and let them pray over him, anointing him with oil in the name of the Lord; And the prayer of faith shall save the sick, and the Lord shall raise him up; and if he have committed sins, they shall be forgiven him.*
>
> — James 5:14–15

Oil was an extremely important commodity in biblical times and was used not only for cooking and fueling lamps, but for external application on wounds, and by extension of those visible benefits, taken internally for illness. In most cases, simple, pure olive oil was used. Fragrance added another dimension to oil, giving it a deeper and more spiritual connotation, and was incorporated in the holy oil for anointing priests and sacred objects, for example. In either case, oil is associated with essential goodness. Psalms 23, which begins, "The Lord is my shepherd; I shall not want. . . ." later says, "Thou anointest my head with oil; my cup runneth over." Psalm 133 says, "How wonderful it is, how pleasant, for God's people to live together in harmony! It is like the precious anointing oil running down from Aaron's head and beard. . . ."

The Christian Church has taken different views on the subject of anointing, with and without added fragrance, and on the subject of incense. Those against its use say it's simply unnecessary, or its use is quasi-magical. One can understand this position to a point, in that fragrance was used in some profusion by religious groups that stood in opposition to Christianity and worshipped other gods with it, such as the Romans, and before them, the "idolaters" who so irked the Jewish prophets by continuing to pay homage to "the queen of heaven." Aiming to distance themselves from these other people, then, early Christians in particular eschewed the use of incense.

When it comes to anointing, the discussion becomes more complex as there are different elements to consider: its use in baptism, confirmation, healing, last rites, ordination of priests, consecration of churches and ritual objects, and the coronation of kings and queens. Over the years, and in different places, opinions have differed over which sacramental practices, if any, should involve the use of oil, and whether they should be perfumed or not. Objections have focused on the thought that nothing physical, such as oil, can represent in any way the blessing of God; God is above the physical, so no physical accoutrements are necessary. Or, as James Pilkington, a sixteenth-century bishop of Durham put it: "What can their holy ashes, holy palms, holy crosses, holy bells, holy creams, relics, moulds, chalice, corporas, fire, candles, beads, or that which is that most holy relic, their oil, wherewith they anoint their shavelings, priests and bishops, do? There is no creature which can give that holiness to another which is in itself; this thing belongs to Christ alone."

Over the centuries there's been endless debate over where to draw the line and, indeed, the Christian Church today finds itself splintered partly as a result of the differences in opinion. The Church of England does not generally anoint, with either plain or perfumed oil, those being baptized; yet a fragrant anointing oil is an important part of the ceremony when an incoming monarch is crowned. On the other hand, the Greek Orthodox Church uses pure olive oil in the sacraments of baptism and holy unction, and a perfumed chrism oil following baptism or when a new convert is received into the church.

Over the years, many commentators have believed that oil, particularly the holy chrism or perfumed oil, in some sense contained the Holy Spirit. But according to Eisenhofer and Lechner in *The Liturgy of the Roman Rite*, oil is merely a symbol for the imparting of grace. In a personal communication, the Reverend Allen Morris informed me that it is not Catholic doctrine "that the oil undergoes substantial change such as does the bread consecrated at the Eucharist." On the subject of the perfumed oil, he says: "The scent of chrism is particularly appropriate for those anointings which lead to the person or object anointed becoming significant of Christ in a particular way. Thus, not only bishops and priests at their ordination, but any person at their baptism, and altars consecrated for their sacred use."

One member of the Russian Orthodox Church, Gillian Crow, has kindly offered her personal interpretation of the use of fragrance in that tradition, as follows:

> As a rule, Orthodox worship aims to be heaven on earth, and expresses the beauty of the fact of God's love. It therefore tries to be beautiful in every possible way, including fragrance. There is nothing in Orthodoxy that is suspicious of beauty. . . . The house of God therefore is expected to be sweet-smelling. . . . Because orthodoxy understands the human being as a unique being of body and soul together, both loved by God, and both destined to rise to eternal life — as demonstrated by the incarnation, life, death, and Resurrection of Jesus Christ, God became human — it insists on the body sharing with the soul in the spiritual life, just as the soul shares with the body in the physical life. Therefore worship and prayer, like every aspect of life, is both a physical and spiritual experience in which body and soul take part. Worship, whether private or public, therefore involves all five senses, of which one is the sense of smell.

There are a variety of opinions regarding the use of fragrance in a spiritual context, no more so than within the Christian tradition. Opinions vary along the whole spectrum, from "It's a pointless indulgence" to "It contains the Holy Spirit." For someone who is inexperienced in the potential effects of aroma, this disparity could be highly confusing. Where there is some hostility to the use of fragrance, this may be because aroma is little understood. For example, essential oils, which are contained in all natural fragrant plant materials, are often very medicinal. When vast clouds of fragrant incense smoke descend on a congregation, some might think, "That'll purify the atmosphere in here," while another person, unaware of the vibrational and medicinal properties, might say, "What a load of superstitious hokum." Similarly, I know essential oils can deeply affect spiritual perception and believe this was one of the reasons fragrance was used in such abundance in ancient, and indeed modern, times.

Others may simply think, "It covers up bad smells," or offer a metaphorical or symbolic explanation for its use. Spirituality is, of course, a personal journey, but in time, perhaps, more credence will be given to the use of aroma in a spiritual context.

ANCIENT GREECE AND ROME

> *Let the rich fumes of od'rous incense fly,*
> *A grateful savour to the powers on high;*
> *The due libation nor neglect to pay,*
> *When evening closes, or when dawns the day.*
> — Hesiod

In Greek mythology, the origin and use of fragrance was attributed to the gods, who lost their monopoly of the secrets when one of Venus's nymphs, Aeone, was indiscreet. When Greek goddesses made an appearance on earth, there was always an associated fragrance, while in their heaven the gods and goddesses enjoyed special wonderful perfumes not available to humans. Worshippers hoped to reach the Greek heaven, the Elysian fields, which were redolent with fragrance, as here described by author Eugene Rimmel:

> In the midst of the Elysian fields they were to find a golden city with emerald ramparts, ivory pavement, and cinnamon gates. Around the walls flowed a river of perfumes one hundred cubits in width, and deep enough to swim in. From this river rose an odorous mist, which enveloped the whole place and shed a refreshing and fragrant dew. There were to be, besides, in this fortunate city, 365 fountains of honey and 500 of the sweetest essences.

No wonder the worship of gods and goddesses was invariably accompanied by sweet fragrance. At home, incense was burned on the thyterion, the incense altar, while at gatherings where animal sacrifice was involved, it was put on an altar along with herbs, flowers, and resins. Vegetarians such as Pythagoras just "sacrificed" plant materials. As there were thousands of Greek gods and goddesses, there were many religious festivals, when fragrant materials were used in great profusion.

The first book entirely dedicated to fragrance, *Concerning Odors*, was written by "the father of botany," Theophrastus, who was born in Lesbos in 370 BCE.

From him and other sources we know the Greeks used, among other fragrances, cassia, cinnamon, cardamom, spikenard, storax, iris, costus, saffron, myrrh, kyperion, ginger-grass, sweet flag, sweet marjoram, lotus, dill, rose, gillyflower, lilies (susinon), myrtle, oil of balanos, bergamot, bay, mint, thyme, hyacinth, violet, and narcissus.

These plants were made into essences and incorporated into oils and unguents using olive, sesame, castor, and linseed oils. Wine was another popular carrier of fragrant material. Apollonius of Herophilia wrote *Treatise on Perfumes*, which listed the best sources of particular ingredients and blends. He lamented the loss of a good source of frankincense "unguent": "Long ago there used to be a most delicious unguent extracted from frankincense at Pergamus, owing to the invention of a certain perfumer of that city, for no one else had ever made it before him; but now none is made there."

The medicinal qualities of aromatic plants were much appreciated at this time, with Criton, Galen, and Hippocrates all advocating the use of fumigations at the time of epidemics. Theophrastus wrote:

> It is to be expected that perfumes should have medicinal properties in view of the virtues of their spices. The effect of plasters and of what some call poultices prove these virtues, since they disperse tumors and abscesses and produce a distinct effect on the body and also its interior parts. If one lays a plaster on his abdomen and breast, he produces fragrant odors in his breath.

Perfumes, with their health-giving properties, were seen as gifts of the gods, and perfumes were in return offered on the altars of worship. At the temples of Venus and the Roman god of medicine, Aesculapius, the recipes of particularly effective essences were inscribed on marble plaques, so the attendants could easily refer to them when healing the sick. According to the Roman author Pliny, in the first century, the plaster of the temple of Minerva, at Elis, had been mixed with saffron by Panaenus, with the result that "even today, if one wets one's thumb with saliva and rubs it on the plaster, the latter still gives off the smell and taste of saffron." Worship was fragrant indeed!

> *The simple savin on the altars smoked,*
> *A laurel sprig the easy gods invoked,*
> *And rich was he whose votive wreath possessed*
> *The lovely violet with sweet flowers dress'd.*
>
> — Ovid

The Romans adopted the Greek practices of using incense in worship, bathing in fragrant water, and massaging with perfumed oils, and took them to the limits. They offered incense not only to their gods but to their living god, the emperor. Their civic baths were of course legendary, comprising the tepidarium, calidarium, sudatorium, and frigidarium, rooms and pools of varying temperature. There was also the unctuarium, where the body could be massaged with perfumed oils. In Rome, the use of rose oil became something of a cult.

The spiritual aspect of fragrance was not ignored, however. Cornelius Agrippa wrote, "If of coriander, smallage, henbane, and hemlock, be made a fume, spirits do presently come together."

THE VEDIC SCRIPTURES

> *There is a Spirit which is mind and life, light and truth and vast spaces.*
> *He contains all works and desires and all perfumes and all tastes. He*
> *enfolds the whole universe, and in silence is loving to all.*
>
> — Chandogya Upanishad

The earliest sacred poetic writings of Hinduism are known as the Vedas, which were completed around 900 BCE. There are four groups of these prayers and hymns: the Rig-Veda, the Sama-Veda, the Yajur-Veda, and the Atharva-Veda. Other religious writings followed, including the Upanishads, Brahmanas, and Puranas. Together, they form the religious writings of Hinduism.

Hinduism is monotheistic, not polytheistic. Although there appear to be many gods and goddesses, they are all aspects of the one god, Brahma, identified with the symbol *OM* and conceptualized now less as a person than as a nonpersonalized divine principle. The Trimurti, or triad of gods, is the first layer of the manifestation of this principle and is composed of Brahma (the creator), Vishnu (the preserver), and Siva (the destroyer). According to the Vedas, their worship should involve burning fires of fragrant woods at the four cardinal points, onto which consecrated oils should be put, while a fragrant grass called kusa is scattered around (possibly *Cymbopogon jwarancusa*, known as "karakusa"). This practice was mentioned in the poem "Sakoontala," written by Kalidasa two thousand years ago, in which the girl of the title is about to be married. Her father speaks:

> Holy flames that gleam around
> Every altar's hallowed ground;
> Holy flames, whose frequent food
> Is the consecrated wood,
> And for whose encircling bed
> Sacred Kusa-grass is spread;
> Holy flames that waft to heaven
> Sweet oblations daily given,
> Mortal guilt to purge away;
> Hear, oh, hear me, when I pray,
> Purify my child this day!

The wives of the Trimurti are the goddesses Sarasvati, Lakshmi, and Sati, although Siva has another wife, who is known by several names, depending on the aspect of herself that is shown, including Parvati and Kali. An aspect of Brahma, or OM, could have many incarnations, and so the god Vishnu is manifested as Rama, Krishna, and Buddha. In this way, with ever-increasing ripples of complexity, with spouses, sons, daughters, lifetimes, and personality aspects, there are literally hundreds of Hindu gods, all manifestations of the one divine principle.

India, the home of Hinduism, is a place where many fragrant plants abound. Fragrance is an integral part of worship, ritual, and ceremony, and has been so for as long as written records can show. Sandalwood is mentioned, for example, in the oldest Vedic scripture, the Nirukta. India has produced certain fragrances for a very long time indeed, including sandalwood, aloeswood, cassia, costus, patchouli, cinnamon, spikenard, rose, jasmine, saffron, turmeric, ginger, camphor, vetiver, cypress, pine, and aniseed, while long-established trade links to the West have ensured an ongoing supply of the Arabic gums and of benzoin from Sumatra and Malaysia to the East. India produces many essential oils not generally used in Western aromatherapy, which derive from the many fragrant flowers growing there, such as pandang, bookool, and kurna. Basil is considered a sacred herb in India, where it is known as tulsi.

The heavens and gods are fragrant, according to the Vedas. There are said to be five heavens, presided over by Brahma, Vishnu, Siva, Kuvera, and Indra, each of which is full of flowers and redolent with fragrance. A blue champac flower is said to grow abundantly in Brahma's heaven, while in Indra's a flower called camalata has a delightful fragrance with the power to grant a person their wishes. Brahma emerged from a lotus flower that grew from the navel of

Vishnu. Kama, the god of love, carries five arrows to pierce the five senses, all tipped with flower blossoms, while Indra is associated with sandalwood. Temples were often partly built of sandalwood, such as the thousand-year-old gates at Somnath.

Incense and essential oils are a central aspect of Hindu worship, with the fragrances of *dhoop* and *dhoona* emanating from countless public temples and private shrines. During the Krishna festivals, a red powder diluted in rose water is splattered over the participants, while during marriage ceremonies, scented oils are thrown into the sacred fire, the *oman*, along with sandalwood incense and other fragrant materials. Fragrant woods and incense are an integral part of the funeral pyre. On the last day of the Hindu year, Divali, sometime during the month of October or November, many rituals are carried out, including the offering of flowers to the gods and goddesses. In some places, impurities are symbolically washed away through the dowsing of water; in wealthy households, rose water and sandalwood are added. Indeed, as anyone who has visited India knows, fragrance is an integral part of daily life, as is spirituality itself.

> *. . . the worship of gods . . . requires the use of auspicious perfumes and*
> *incense; it contributes to the pleasures of men; it leads to the attainment*
> *of the three ends of human life (that is, religious merit, worldly prosperity*
> *and sensual enjoyment). . . .*
>
>   — Gangadhara, Gandhasara, c. 750 CE

ISLAM AND ARABIA

> *It has been given to me to love three things in your base world: women,*
> *perfumes and prayer, but the apple of my eye is prayer.*
>
>   — Muhammad (Hadith)

Muhammad, the prophet of Islam, was very fond of aromatics. Through his close association with traders, he had access to spices and resins and would have known about their healing and other properties. It is said, for example, that a pustule on his finger was cured by the application, in a bandage, of *Acorus calamus*, sweet flag, an aromatic perennial. In his time too, teeth were kept clean with *Salvadora persica*, the twigs of which are cut to make a natural brush with built-in toothpaste. According to the early eleventh-century Arabian doctor and philosopher Avicenna, Muhammad appreciated "excellent odors" because "they fortify the senses. And when the senses are strong, the thoughts are precise and their conclusions upright. When, on the other hand, the senses become weak, thoughts become unbalanced and their conclusions confused." Avicenna traveled a great deal and wrote many books, including *Canon Medicinae*, a huge reference book that was invaluable to many Arab and European medical students for centuries. He is also credited with inventing the first "modern" distilling apparatus, capable of extracting essential oils from flower petals. A hundred years ago in France, a still was called *al-embicm*, showing its Arabic origin.

Muhammad was born around 570 CE, at which time the Arabs were already great traders. He moved from Mecca to Medina in 622, spreading the message of the Koran, and from 661 onward, Islam was carried by the Umayyad caliphs to Spain in the west, and along the northern coast of Africa to eastern Turkey, Persia, and as far east as the Indus valley. The Arab traders ventured even farther, overland to China and across the Sahara Desert to West Africa, and by sailing in *dhows* to East Africa and Zanzibar, and Southeast Asia. All along the way, they traded in a great variety of aromatics.

The fragrances most associated with Muhammad are rose, myrtle, violet, and henna-flower. Muhammad is reported to have said, "When I was taken up to heaven, some of my sweat fell on the earth, and from it sprang the rose, and whoever would smell my scent, let him have the rose." The Arabs are said to have preserved roses by putting blooms in a pottery jar, sealing the lid with clay, burying it in the ground until needed, then taking the blooms out and sprinkling them with water — at which point they sprung back to life.

Over the years a great deal has been written about the fragrances to be found in the Muslim paradise, which are said to be fabulous, although the Koran itself refers only to "gardens under which rivers flow." No doubt the association of fragrance with heaven has grown from the prophet's own appreciation of fragrance and, indeed, from the Arab people's love of perfumes in general. It is said, after all, that in heaven you will find all that you most desire.

Centuries before Muhammad was born, Arab traders were supplying the great civilizations of Egypt and Mesopotamia with the fragrant materials that grew in their lands, such as frankincense, olibanum, myrrh, jasmine, and rose. From the ancient Greeks they learned the elements of chemistry and medicine, which they greatly further developed. Indeed, the Arabs between the sixth and eleventh centuries were the repository of much wisdom in medicine and science and can truly be called the cultural bridge between the old civilizations and the new one that grew from the Italian Renaissance period.

BUDDHA OF THE SACRED TREE

This supreme incense, the aroma of pure moral conduct,
We bless with meditation, mantra and mudra.
As this glorious fragrance pervades the Buddha realms,
May an ocean of Buddhas be delighted!

                              — Tibetan prayer

Buddha was born as Prince Siddhartha Gautama in what is now northern India or Nepal, in the sixth or seventh century BCE. In the first century BCE, the first canonical texts were written, in Pali, an ancient Indian language, so for at least five hundred years the teachings of Buddha, and details of his life, were handed down orally. It's now generally accepted that Buddha grew up in great royal luxury, unaware of the travails of life, married at sixteen, and thirteen years later had a son, an event that awakened in him thoughts of life, death, and the meaning of it all. He was determined to renounce his sheltered life with its attendant pleasures, and took to a wandering life, through which he hoped to find a panacea for the vicissitudes of life.

For six years he followed the course of great self-denial, fasting and meditating and seeking wisdom from the Hindu gurus he met along the way. Unsatisfied with this course of action, he decided on "the Middle Way," neither indulgence nor denial. He decided the answer was to be found within his own consciousness, and settled under an Indian fig tree, a pipal, or bodhi, tree, and began to meditate. After four weeks, some say seven, he attained enlightenment. The Four Noble Truths of Buddhism are: life involves suffering; we suffer because we desire; to end desire means the end of suffering; and this can be accomplished by following the "eightfold path" — right views, right aspiration, right speech, right conduct, right livelihood, right effort, right mindfulness, and right contemplation.

Buddhism spread southward, to Sri Lanka, Burma, Vietnam, Cambodia, Thailand, Malaysia, Indonesia, and the Philippines, and north and east to Tibet, China, Korea, and Japan, while it declined in India itself. It has often taken on the flavor of other, older religious teachings encountered along the way, many of which also involved the offering of fragrant material. Today at Buddhist shrines, huge amounts of incense are burned before images of the Buddha, in the form of burning woods, resins, or incense sticks. In China, the woods of camphor, pine, and sandalwood are commonly used, along with fragrant spices.

Camphor wood was once the material preferred to make the rosaries used by Buddhist monks and nuns, and also the boxes or chests that held the sacred texts, the Sutras. Worshippers often light three incense sticks, which are held in their hands while the smoke is blown three times, before putting the incense down and placing the palms of the hands together, in prayer. In Japan, ground incense is carried around in little boxes, from where a small amount can be placed on the hands and inhaled while making a prayer.

In Buddhist practice, incense is symbolic of several ideas. The sweetness of the aroma signifies pure moral conduct, delightful in the same way as is the practice of giving up those things that are damaging or hurtful. It represents, metaphorically, the giving, the generosity of correct Buddhist practice, the overcoming of greed and selfishness. As the smoke rises and moves through the air, it can also be seen as the Buddhist teachings spreading across the world. Incense is also appreciated as being simply pleasant, for those offering it and for others around.

In Tibet, Buddhism encountered and became mingled with the earlier folk religion, Bon, in which offerings and prayers were presented to ancestral spirits, family spirits, and the deceased. Deities were seen to reside in mountains or plains, in the soil or in trees, rocks, or rivers. According to Tucci in *The Religions of Tibet*, "None of the local communities was ready to renounce its old protective gods. . . . Admitted into the new religion as guardians of the Law, they now punish each violation of the Law or transgression of the Buddhist vow."

Each morning in Tibet incense is offered, most usually in the form of juniper, although other fragrant trees and shrubs such as *bu lu*, "rhododendron," and *stag pa*, "birch," are also used. The smoke of the offering is said to be purifying and atoning. There are three types of juniper in Tibet, *Juniperus pseudosabina*, known as "the central Asian juniper," *Juniperus squamosa*, a low shrub similar to *Juniperus communis*, and *Juniper excelsa*, the "pencil cedar" tree that covers much of the Himalayan mountains and is considered sacred. This cypresslike tree produces berries (*shug 'bras*) that are burned as incense, and in the earlier Bon tradition, were once used as a narcotic to help induce trance.

In every Tibetan home there is a small altar, possibly several, in which incense, juniper, tsampa, dried fruits, and other offerings are burned. Juniper branches are burned in the high stone and earth stoves (*bsangs-thab*) kept on every flat Tibetan roof for that purpose. On special occasions, the ritual would be somewhat more elaborate, as described by Dorje Yudon Yuthok in *House of the Turquoise Roof*:

To make this special offering, slightly green juniper branches were burned along with two or three spoonfuls of barley mixed with butter, which were added before lighting the fire. When the fire was smoldering, another small juniper branch was dipped into a bowl of clean water and used to sprinkle the flames three times while the mantra, "Om Ah Hum," was repeated each time. The ceremony purified the offering of incense and produced a very pleasant fragrance.

TAOISM AND CHINESE TRADITION

Cling to the Unity.
— Taoist maxim

Taoism is said to have started with Lao Tzu in the sixth century BCE, although the philosophy may in fact have developed two hundred years later. Indeed, the origins of Taoism are uncertain, with Joseph Campbell referring to Lao Tzu as "a *complete* mirage" and a "mythical sage." Nevertheless, there are some very ancient texts referring to a Lao Tzu, which means "old master," and a philosophy, Taoism, which is about "going with the flow" of nature and recognizing the balance between the opposites, including yin and yang.

So deeply did the ancient Chinese wish to "go" with nature, they spent a great deal of time trying to emulate it in that they sought the eternal. Immortality, or at least achieving a ripe old age, became something of a preoccupation, with the literature full of heroic journeys and adventures undertaken to find various herbs, fruits, and fungi of immortality. As well as many mythical plants, various real plants were considered to have "soul substance," or the "essence of life," including cassia, pine, cypress, and camphor.

The transformational aspects of nature were a source of great wonder, particularly the seasons. Incense, with its ability to change from one form to another — fragrant material to smoke — came to be seen as representative of the Tao and was a vital component in Taoist worship. Each service still begins with lighting the incense burner (*fa-lu*), and at the end of worship, the incense burner is again replenished (*fu-lu*).

SHINTO AND THE JAPAN TRADITION

Plants are used in ceremony because God is invited to join us through the plant.... Everything in the beginning had a good smell. Even things today

*we consider bad smells, were good. In ancient times everything smelt
good — all of life. All souls enjoyed the smells, every day. For example, I
make fire and I feel the smell of fire. The smell of fire, not the wood. The
actual fire has a smell. The fire is a kind of ceremony.*

> — Mikinosuke Kakisaha, Shinto high priest,
> Tenkawa Temple, 1997

Shinto, a uniquely Japanese religion from the eighth century BCE, predates the arrival of Buddhism. Joseph Campbell describes it: "Shinto, at root, is a religion not of sermons but of awe: which is a sentiment that may or may not produce words, but in either case goes beyond them. Not a 'grasp of the conception of spirit,' but a sense of its ubiquity." Shinto does not follow a set moral code, but is moralistic in recognizing the difference between doing good and evil, of being pure and impure.

Perhaps because Shinto so deeply appreciates and venerates the intrinsic beauty in the living world, the Japanese have developed several unique art forms involving natural materials. There are stunning Zen Buddhist gardens, which owe more to the Japanese reverence of nature than to Buddhism itself. The trees, shrubs, and stones are arranged with quiet, purposeful reverence. Similarly in Japan, flower arranging has been elevated to an art form appreciative of every angle of every stem, highlighting the glorious radiance of every flower. Also, Japan has made the appreciation of incense into an art, known as *Koh-do*, the incense ceremony. A few fragrant woods are chosen, and by means of a guessing game, participants inhale the aroma of each in turn, slowly and purposefully appreciating each unique aroma. These three unique Japanese art forms are about the development of the senses, the awe of nature, and have Shinto at their heart.

Incense, *koh*, is widely used in Japan, in worship at home and at Buddhist shrines, although Japan itself does not produce most materials used, which have to be imported. The main ingredients of koh are *jinkoh* (aloeswood), of which there are several varieties including the very expensive *kyara*, sandalwood, ginger, cassia, cinnamon, benzoin, camphor, clove, frankincense, star anise, patchouli, myrrh, *kansho* (an East Indian rhizome), *rei-ryokoh* (an Asian mint), and the root of a Chinese plant, *haiso*. One indigenous ingredient is the bark of *Cercidiphyllum japonicum*.

Incense comes in various forms. As well as the familiar incense sticks, there are long-burning incense coils, incense balls, incense cones, chopped mixtures for putting on hot ashes in altars, and *nioi-bukuro*, little cloth or paper sachets of ground incense used to fragrance clothing, rooms, and drawers, or hung around the neck. They were once widely believed to offer protection from bad luck. Ground incense is also carried in small boxes, from where it can be rubbed on the hands before prayer.

At Shinto shrines, incense or piles of fragrant wood and branches are burned so worshippers can direct the profuse smoke over themselves and others. This practice was once ubiquitous all over the world in ancient and historical times, and is not unique to Shinto. But it is perhaps unusual today in being such an important part of organized official religious practice, and is indicative of Shinto's ancient roots.

THE NATIVE AMERICAN NATIONS

> *This smoke from the sweet grass will rise up to You, and will spread throughout the universe; its fragrance will be known by the wingeds, the four-leggeds, and the two-leggeds...*
>
> — High Hollow Horn,
> *The Sacred Pipe*

To the Native American nations, spirit resides not only in people and animals, but in the earth, sky, stars, trees, herbs, flowers, and rocks. The whole of living nature has the same ultimate spiritual source and is deserving of respect. Our living in harmony with nature brings out the best in it, and us.

In *Gift of Power*, Sioux medicine man Archie Fire Lame Deer recounts an event he witnessed one day involving his grandfather, a Lakota medicine man and spiritual leader:

> The stroke had left one of Grandma Lizzie's sides paralyzed, and she had lost the power of speech. Grandpa had someone heat a rock over a fire while he and I went to pick certain herbs that were needed for the healing. . . . Grandpa took his buffalo horn, which was his most powerful medicine, and went into Lizzie's room. He wrapped her in a buffalo robe, put the heated rock under the small of her back, and purified her with cedar incense, using his eagle wing to fan the fragrant smoke toward her. . . [he sang] sacred songs at Lizzie's bedside . . . half an hour after the doctoring began, Grandma Lizzie came out of the house. She was walking around and chatting as if nothing had happened.

There are many spiritual practices among the Native American nations, which differ from place to place, although common to many are smudging, the medicine wheel, the sacred pipe ceremony, the sweat lodge, the vision quest, and the sun dance. The vision quest is a personal journey of spiritual discovery involving meditation and fasting, while the sun dance is a communal ceremony of giving thanks.

The sweat lodge is a tentlike building, with a roof made of bent branches covered with hides or other material. At its center is a collection of red-hot rocks, on which water and herbs are placed, creating very hot steam. Some sweat lodges are single sex, either male or female; some are mixed. The one I attended on a Cree reservation was a mixed lodge of about sixteen people, men on one side, women on the other. It started around 10:30 PM, and although a large fire was kept burning outside, because the flaps were kept tightly shut inside it was completely dark. The darkness allows you to see, not with your eyes and logical mind, but with your spirit.

To say it was hot would be a major understatement, but despite being uncomfortable at times, the heat was also releasing: you have to "let go." The smell of the sage burning on the hot rocks filled the humid atmosphere, and as each person in turn spoke their prayers out loud and gave thanks, the drums and rattles added their special tones. As Archie Fire Lame Deer writes, "The sweat lodge becomes the universe, the whole world concentrated in a tiny hut." In his nation, three herbs are used during the *Inipi*, the sweat lodge: sweetgrass, sage, and cedar. A bundle of sage might also be used to sprinkle water on the hot stones.

It is difficult to overestimate the importance of fragrant herbs and trees to the spiritual ceremonies of Native American nations. They are also a crucial ingredient in personal medicine bundles, or spiritual talismans. The United States is such a vast continent with various landscapes and flora, one would expect there to be differences from place to place in the plant materials used in ritual. Besides those already mentioned, spruce, pine, and juniper are also important.

> . . . I remain undaunted, for I dwell within my Spirit that is filled with the
> heady essence of Sage, Cedar, and Sweetgrass, and with my head held
> high do I walk into the light that illuminates my new trail.
>
> — Mary Summer Rain

Appendix One

SAFETY DATA

Not all natural plants or plant products are beneficial to health. Deadly nightshade can be poisonous, and stinging nettles sting. The following essential oils should NOT be used under any circumstances:

Bitter Almond
Boldo Leaf
Calamus
Horseradish
Jaborandi Leaf
Mugwort
Mustard
Pennyroyal
Rue

Sassafras
Savin
Southernwood
Tansy
Thuja
Wintergreen
Wormseed
Wormwood
Yellow Camphor

Essential oils are highly concentrated plant essences and should not be taken orally unless you are under medical supervision.

If you have sensitive skin or allergic reactions to aromatic materials, you should always do a skin test twenty-four hours before using them.

Some essential oils have been documented as causing photosensitivity and should not be applied to the skin before exposure to the sun. Of those mentioned in this book, oils that may fall into this category are among the citrus group — especially bergamot — and angelica. See also Special Care, page 40.

PREGNANCY

In pregnancy, the usual quantities of any essential oil should be reduced by at least half. Certain essential oils should be avoided altogether during pregnancy or when breast-feeding. These are:

Aniseed	Cumin	Parsley Seed
Basil	Fennel	Peppermint
Bay	Hops	Pimento Berry
Birch	Hyssop	Rosemary
Black Pepper	Juniper	Sage
Cedarwood	Mace	Spikenard
Cinnamon	Marjoram	Tarragon
Cistus	Myrrh	Thyme
Clary Sage	Nutmeg	Valerian
Clove	Oregano	

Appendix Two

Suppliers

For energetically pure essential oils suitable for the purposes outlined in *Aromatherapy for the Soul*, contact the following sources, which supply essential oils internationally.

Valerie Worwood
PO Box 38
Romford, Essex RM1 DN, England
www.valerieworwood.com

High-quality essential oils, Mother Essences, Aroma-Genera oils and Be-spoke Essential Blends

Earthgarden
Essential Oil and Herbal Dispensary
Valerie Worwood Essential Oils and Products
2 Fairview Parade, Mawney Road,
Romford, Essex, RM7 7HH, England

Telephone and Fax (00 44) 1708 722633
www.earthgarden.co.uk

Bibliography

Abraham, Ralph, Terence McKenna, and Rupert Sheldrake. *Trialogues at the Edge of the West*. Santa Fe: Bear and Co., 1992.

Ackerman, Diane. *A Natural History of the Senses*. New York: Random House, 1993.

Adams, George, and Olive Whicher. *The Plant Between Sun and Earth*. London: Steiner Press, 1980.

Afnan, S. M. *Avicenna: His Life and Works*. London: Greenwood Press, 1958.

Alder, Vera Stanley. *The Finding of the Third Eye*. London: Ryder and Co., 1982.

Ali, Abdallah Yousuf, trans. *The Glorious Kur'an*. Lahore, Pakistan, 1934.

Alon, Azaria. *Flowers and Trees of the Holy Land*. Jerusalem: Palphot, n.d.

Andrews, Ted. *Sacred Sounds*. St. Paul: Llewellyn Publications, 1993.

Arcier, Micheline. *Aromatherapy: Health and Beauty Care with Massage and Essential Oils*. London: Hamlyn, 1990.

Ash, David A. *The New Science of the Spirit*. London: The College of Psychic Studies, 1995.

Avigad, Brakha, and Avinoam Danin. *Flowers of Jerusalem*. Tel Aviv: E. Lewin-Epstein-Modan Publishers, 1977.

Babbitt, Edwin D. *The Principles of Light and Colour*. Secaucus, NJ: Citadel Press, 1967.

Bach, Edward. *Heal Thyself*. Saffron Walden, UK: C. W. Daniel Co., 1982.

Bailey, Alice. *Esoteric Healing*. London: Lucis Press, 1984.

Balfour, John Hutton. *The Plants of the Bible*. London: T. Nelson and Sons, 1885.

Barker, Margaret. *The Lost Prophet*. London: SPCK, 1988.

Beattie, James Herries. *Traditional Lifeways of the Southern Maori*. Dunedin, New Zealand: University of Otago Press, 1994.

Becker, Robert O., and Gary Salden. *The Body Electric*. New York: William Morrow, 1987.

Bennett, J. G. *Gurdjieff: A Very Great Enigma*. York Beach, Maine: Samuel Weiser, 1984.

Benor, Daniel J. "Survey of Spiritual Healing Research." *Complementary Medical Research*, 4, no. 1 (September 1990).

Benor, Daniel J. "Survey of Spiritual Healing Research." *Healing Research*, vols. 1 and 2, Munich: Helix Verlag GmbH, 1993.

Birren, Faber. *Colour Psychology and Colour Therapy*. Secaucus, NJ: Citadel Press, 1961.

Boeser, Knut, ed. *The Elixirs of Nostradamus*. London: Bloomsbury, 1995.

Book of Mormon, and the Doctrine of Covenants. Salt Lake City: The Church of Jesus Christ of Latter Day Saints, 1981.

Borghia, Anthony. *Life in the World Unseen*. London: Psychic Press, 1981.

Brunton, Dr. Paul. *A Search in Secret Egypt*. London: Ryder and Co., 1980.

Bruyere, Rosalyn L. *Wheels of Light*. New York: Simon and Schuster, 1994.

Budge, E. A. Wallace. *The Divine Origin of the Craft of the Herbalist*. New York: Dover Publications Inc., 1996.

Buhner, Stephen Harrod. *Sacred Plant Medicine: Explorations in the Practice of Indigenous Herbalism*. Boulder, Colo.: Roberts Rinehart, 1996.

Burr, Harold Saxton. *Blueprint for Immortality: The Electric Patterns of Life*. Saffron Walden, UK: C. W. Daniel Co., 1972.

Callcott, Maria. *A Scripture Herbal*. London: Longman, Brown, Green and Longmans, 1842.

Campbell, Joseph. *Occidental Mythology*. London: Arkana/Penguin, 1991.

———. *Oriental Mythology*. London: Arkana/Penguin, 1991.

———. *The Way of the Seeded Earth*. Vol. 2. New York: Harper & Row, 1989.

Case, E. M. *Odour of Sanctity*. Exeter, UK: private publication, n.d.

Chapman, Rev. David M. *The Fragrance of the Spirit*. Exeter: The Methodist Sacramental Fellowship, 1997.

Charles, R. H., trans. *The Book of Enoch*. London: SPCK, 1997.

Classen, C., D. Howes, and Anthony Synnot. *Aroma, the Cultural History of Smell*. London: Routledge, 1994.

Coats, Callum. *Living Energies*. Bath, UK: Gateway Books, 1996.

Connolly, David. *In Search of Angels*. New York: Perigee Books, 1993.

Cooper, Rev. Henry. *Holy Unction*. London: The Guild of St. Raphael, 1966.

Copen, Bruce. *A Rainbow of Health*. Haywards Heath, UK: Acaedemic Publications, 1984.

Cotterell, Arthur. *The Encyclopaedia of Ancient Civilisations*. London: Macmillan, 1983.

Cowan, Eliot. *Plant Spirit Medicine*. Columbus, NC: Swan Raven & Co., 1995.

Davidson, Gustav. *A Dictionary of Angels*. New York: The Free Press, 1994.

Davidson, John. *Radiation*. Saffron Walden, UK: C. W. Daniel Co., 1986.

———. *Subtle Energy*. Saffron Walden, UK: C. W. Daniel Co., 1987.

———. *The Web of Life*. Saffron Walden, UK: C. W. Daniel Co., 1988.

Davis, Richard H. *Ritual in an Oscillating Universe*. Princeton University Press, 1991.

Dawood, N. J., trans. *The Koran*. Harmondsworth, UK: Penguin, 1983.

Des Roches, Christian. *Tutankhamen*. London: Michael Joseph, 1969.

De Waal, M. *Medicinal Herbs in the Bible*. York Beach, ME: Samuel Weiser, 1984.

Devereux, Paul. *The Long Trip: A Prehistory of Psychedelia*. New York: Penguin/Arkana, 1997.

Dossey, Larry. *Healing Words*. San Francisco: HarperCollins, 1997.

———. *Prayer Is Good Medicine*. San Francisco: HarperCollins, 1996.

Dudley, Martin, and Geoffrey Rowell. *The Oil of Gladness, Anointing in the Christian Tradition*. London: SPCK, 1993.

Dumitrescu, Ion, and Julian N. Kenyon. *Electrographic Imaging in Medicine and Biology*. Sudbury, UK: Neville Spearman, 1983.

Elliott, Maurice. *Spiritualism in the Old Testament*. London: Psychic Press, 1938.

Endicott, K. *Batek Negrito Religion: The World-View and Rituals of a Hunting and Gathering People of Peninsular Malaysia*. Oxford: Clarendon Press, 1979.

Evans-Wentz, W. Y. *Cuchama and Sacred Mountains*. Athens, OH: Swallow Press, 1981.

Fire Lame Deer, Archie. *Gift of Power*. Santa Fe: Bear and Co., 1992.

Fox, Matthew, and Rupert Sheldrake. *The Physics of Angels*. San Francisco: Harper-Collins, 1996.

Fox, Rev. A. H. Purcell. *A Little Book about Holy Unction*. London: The Guild of St. Raphael, 1962.

Frazer, James George. *The Golden Bough*. New York: Viking Penguin, 1998.

Gerber, Richard. *Vibrational Medicine*. Santa Fe: Bear and Co., 1988.

Gerbert, Grohmann. *The Plant*. Vols. 1 and 2. Kimburton, PA: Biodynamic Farming and Gardening Association, 1989.

Gimbel, Theo. *Healing through Colour*. Saffron Walden, UK: C. W. Daniel Co., 1985.

Ginzberg, Louis. *Legends of the Bible*. Philadelphia: The Jewish Publication Society of America, 1978.

Gonen, Rivka. *Biblical Holy Places*. London: A. & C. Black, 1987.

Gooch, Stan. *Cities of Dreams*. London: Aulis Books, 1995.

Greber, Johannes. *Communication with the Spirit World of God*. Teaneck, NJ: Johannes Greber Memorial Foundation, 1979.

Green, Celia, and Charles McCreery. *Apparitions*. Oxford: Institute of Psycho Physical Research, 1995.

Guirdham, Arthur. *A Foot in Both Worlds*. Saffron Walden, UK: C. W. Daniel Co., 1991.

Gurudas. *Gem Elixirs and Vibrational Healing*. Vols. 1 and 2. Boulder, Colo.: Cassandra Press, 1986.

Halevi, Helen. *Reiki: Hawayo Takata's Story*. Olney, MD: Archedigm, 1990.

Halevi, Z'ev ben Shimon. *Kabbalah*. London: Thames and Hudson, 1992.

Hareuveni, Nogah. *Ecology in the Bible*. Jerusalem: Neot Kedumim, 1974.

———. *The Emblem of the State of Israel*. Jerusalem: Neot Kedumim, 1988.

Hay, R. K. M., and P. G. Waterman, eds. *Volatile Oil Crops: Their Biology, Biochemistry, and Production*. London: Longman Group UK, 1993.

Head, Joseph, and Sylvia Cranston. *Reincarnation: The Phoenix Fire Mystery*. Pasadena, Calif.; Theosophical University Press, 1994.

Hepper, F. Nigel. *Illustrated Encyclopaedia of Bible Plants*. London: Three's Company, 1992.

———. *Pharaoh's Flowers*. London: HMSO, 1990.

———. *Planting a Bible Garden*. London: HMSO, 1991.

Herodotus. *The History*. Trans. Henry Cary. Buffalo, New York: Prometheus Books, 1992.

Hitti, P. K. *History of the Arabs*. London: Macmillan, 1951.

Holy Bible. London: Collins, 1958.

Holy Bible: New International Version. London: Hodder & Stoughton, 1985.

Holy Scriptures: According to the Masoretic Text. Vols. 1 and 2. Philadelphia: The Jewish Publication Society of America, 1976.

Howell, S. *Society and Cosmos: Chewong of Peninsular Malaysia*. Oxford: Oxford University Press, 1984.

Hunt, Roland. *Fragrant and Radiant Healing Symphony*. Rochford, UK: C. W. Daniel Co., n.d.

Hunt, Valerie V. *The Infinite Mind: The Science of Human Vibrations*. Malibu, Calif.: Malibu Publishing Co., 1995.

Hurnard, Hannah. *Mountains of Spices*. Eastbourne, UK: Kingsway Publications, 1985.

Hutchens, Alma R. *Indian Herbology of North America*. Windsor, Ontario: Merco, 1986.

Jayjakar, Pupul. *The Earth Mother*. Harmondsworth, UK: Penguin, 1989.

Jigmenorbu, Thubten, and Colin Turnbull. *Tibet: Its History, Religion & People*. London: Penguin, 1983.

Karagulla, Shafica, and Dora van Gelder Kunz. *The Chakras and the Human Energy Fields*. Wheaton, Ill.: Quest Books, 1991.

Kennett, Frances. *History of Perfume*. London: George G. Harrap & Co., 1975.

Khan, Hazratinayat. *The Mysticism of Sound and Music*. Boston: Shambhala, 1996.

Leadbeater, C. W. *The Perfume of Egypt and Other Weird Stories*. Aydar, Madras, India, 1911.

Le Guerer, Annick. *Scent: The Mysterious and Essential Powers of Smell*. London: Chatto & Windus, 1993.

Loehr, Rev. Franklin. *The Power of Prayer on Plants*. New York: Doubleday, 1959.

Long, Asphodel P. *In a Chariot Drawn by Lions*. London: Women's Press, 1992.

Lucretius. *On the Nature of Things, Book 3* Indianapolis: Hackett, 2001.

Mackenzie, Donald A. *China and Japan: Myths and Legends*. London: Senate/Studio Editions, 1994.

Maclean, Dorothy. *To Hear the Angels Sing*. New York: Lindisfarne Press, 1990.

Mallasz, Gitta. *Talking with Angels*. Einsiedeln, Switzerland: Daimon Verlag, 1992.

Manniche, Lise. *An Ancient Egyptian Herbal*. London: British Museum Publications, 1989.

Mascaro, Juan, trans. *The Bhagavad Gita*. Harmondsworth, UK: Penguin, 1970.

Maury, Marguerite. *Guide to Aromatherapy: The Secret of Life and Youth*. Saffron Walden, UK: C. W. Daniel Co., 1989.

McKenzie, Dan. *Aromatics and the Soul*. London: William Heinemann, 1923.

Mernissi, Fatima. *Women in Moslem Paradise*. New Delhi: Kali for Women, 1988.

Miller, J. Innes. *The Spice Trade of the Roman Empire*. Oxford: Oxford University Press, 1988.

Moldenke, Harold N., and L. Alma. *Plants of the Bible*. New York: Dover Publications, 1986.

Moody, Raymond A., Jr. *Reflections of Life after Life*. New York: Bantam Books, 1978.

Mookerjee, Ajit. *Kundalini: The Arousal of the Inner Energy*. London: Thames and Hudson, 1983.

Moolenburgh, H. C. *A Handbook of Angels*. Saffron Waldon, UK: C. W. Daniel Co., 1988.

———. *Meeting with Angels*. Saffron Waldon, UK: C. W. Daniel Co., 1993.

Morita, Kiyoko. *The Book of Incense*. Tokyo: Kodansha International, 1992.

Morris, Edwin T. *Fragrance: The Story of Perfume from Cleopatra to Chanel*. New York: E. T. Morris & Co., 1984.

Moskvitin, Jirij. *Essay on the Origin of Thought*. Athens, Ohio: Ohio University Press, 1974.

Murphey, Edith van Allen. *Indian Uses of Native Plants*. Glenwood: Meyer Books, 1990.

Mutma, Credo Vusamazulu. *My People: Writings of a Zulu Witchdoctor*. Harmondsworth, UK: Penguin, 1977.

Myss, Caroline. *Anatomy of the Spirit*. New York: Harmony Books, 1996.

Neumann, Erich. *The Great Mother*. London: Routledge and Kegan Paul, 1963.

Niazi, H. M. *The Egyptian Prescription*. Cairo: Elias Modern Press, 1988.

Oldfield, Harry, and Roger Coghill. *The Dark Side of the Brain*. Shaftsbury, UK: Element Books, 1988.

Ono, Sokyo. *Shinto: The Kami Way*. Boston: Charles E. Tuttle Co., 1994.

Ouseley, S. G. J. *The Power of the Rays*. Romford, UK: L. N. Fowler & Co., 1976.

Pagels, Elaine. *The Gnostic Gospels*. New York: Random House, 1989.

Paulson, Genieve Lewis. *Kundalini and the Chakras*. St. Paul: Llewellyn Publications, 1997.

Pellant, Chris. *The Complete Book of Rocks and Minerals*. London: Dorling Kindersley, 1995.

Pendell, Dale. *Pharmako-Poeia, Plant Powers, Poisons, and Herbcraft*. San Francisco: Mercury House, 1995.

Pert, Candace B. *Molecules of Emotions*. New York: Scribner, 1997.

Piesse, G. W. Septimus. *The Art of Perfumery*. London: Longman Brown Green Longmans and Roberts, 1856.

Plummer, Charles. *Lives of Irish Saints*. Oxford: Oxford University Press, 1997.

Post, George E. *The Botanical Geography of Palestine*. N.p.: private publication, 1888.

Prabhupada, His Divine Grace A. A. C. Bhaktivedanti, Swami. *Coming Back: The Science of Reincarnation*. Sydney: ISKCON, 1982.

Rain, Mary Summer. *Phantoms Afoot*. Donning Co., 1989.

————. *Spirit Song*. Norfolk, Va.: Hampton Roads Publishing Co., 1985.

Ratsch, Dr. Christian. *The Dictionary of Sacred and Magical Plants*. Translated by John Baker. Bridport, UK: Prism Press, 1992.

Reed, A. W. *Aboriginal Myths*. French's Forest, Australia: Reed Books, 1987.

Rimmel, Eugene. *The Book of Perfumes*, 5th ed. London: Chapman and Hall, 1867.

Rinpoche, Sogyal. *The Tibetan Book of Living and Dying*. San Francisco: HarperCollins, 1994.

Roberts, Jane. *The Nature of the Psyche*. San Rafael, Calif.: Amber Allen, 1996.

Robinson, H. Wheeler. *The Christian Experience of the Holy Spirit*. London: Fontana, 1962.

Ross, Dr. A. C. *Mitakuye Oyasin*. Denver: Bear and Co., 1993.

Ross, Hugh McGregor, trans. *The Gospel of St. Thomas*. Shaftsbury, UK: Element Books, 1991.

————. *Thirty Essays on the Gospel of Thomas*. Shaftsbury, UK: Element Books, 1990.

Rossbach, Sarah. *Feng Shui*. London: Hutchinson, 1984.

Scott, Ian. *The Luscher Colour Test*. London: Pan Books, 1983.

Shepsut, Asia. *Journey of the Priestess*. London: Aquarian/Thorsons, 1993.

Shewell-Cooper, W. E. *Plants, Flowers, and Herbs of the Bible*. New Canaan, Conn.: Keats Publishing, 1988.

Shrii Shrii Ananda Murti. *Beyond the Superconscious Mind*. Calcutta: Ananda Marga, 1987.

Smith, E. Lester, V. Wallace Slater, and Gerard Reilly. *The Field of Occult Chemistry*. London: Theosophical Publishing House, 1934.

Snellgrove, Brian. *The Unseen Self*. Saffron Waldon, UK: C. W. Daniel Co., 1996.

Stein, R. *Tibetan Civilization*. Palo Alto, Calif.: Stanford University Press, 1972.

Steiner, Rudolph. *Manifestations of Karma*. London: Rudolph Steiner Press, 1995.

————. *Nature Spirits*. London: Rudolph Steiner Press, 1995.

Stone, Robert B. *The Secret Life of Your Cells*. Atglen, PA: Schiffer Publishing, 1989.

Stonehouse, Julia. *Idols to Incubators: Reproduction Theory through the Ages*. London: Scarlet Press, 1994.

Sylvia, Claire, and William Novak. *A Change of Heart*. New York: Warner Books, 1998.

Szekely, Edmond Bordeaux, trans. *The Gospel of the Essenes*. Saffron Walden, UK: C. W. Daniel Co., 1993.

Talbot, Michael. *Mysticism and the New Physics*. New York: Viking Penguin, 1993.

Tansley, David V. *The Raiment of Light*. London: Routledge and Kegan Paul, 1984.

Thiering, Barbara. *Jesus the Man*. London: Corgi Books, 1993.

Thompson, C. J. S. *The Mystery and Lure of Perfume*. London: John Lane The Bodley Head, n.d.

Tompkins, Peter. *The Secret Life of Nature*. San Francisco: HarperCollins, 1997.

Tucci, G. *The Religions of Tibet*. London: Routledge and Kegan Paul, 1980.

Valnet, Jean. *The Practice of Aromatherapy*. Saffron Walden, UK: C. W. Daniel Co., 1986.

Vogel, Virgil J. *American Indian Medicine*. Norman: University of Oklahoma Press, 1986.

Von Hagen, Victor W. *The Ancient Sun Kingdoms of the Americas*. N.p., 1957.

Walker, Barbara G. *The Woman's Encyclopaedia of Myths and Secrets*. San Francisco: Harper & Row, 1983.

Watson, Lyall. *The Biology of Death*. London: Hodder and Stoughton, 1987.

Weiss, Brian L. *Many Lives, Many Masters*. New York: Simon and Schuster, 1988.

————. *Through Time into Healing*. London: Piatkus, 1995.

Wesley, John. *Primitive Physic*. London: Wesley's Chapel, 1997 (reprint of 18th-century edition).

White, John. *The Meeting of Science and Spirit*. New York: Paragon House, 1990.

Whitman, John. *The Psychic Power of Plants*. London: Star Books/W. H. Allen, 1975.

Wilkinson, Sir J. Gardner. *The Ancient Egyptians — Their Life and Customs*. London: Bracken Books, 1988.

Wilson, Michael. *What Is Colour?* Stourbridge, UK: Goethean Science Foundation, 1983.

Woolger, Roger J. *Other Lives, Other Selves*. Wellingborough, UK: Thorsons Publishing Group, 1990.

Worwood, Valerie Ann. *The Fragrant Mind*. Novato, Calif.: New World Library, 1996.

————. *The Complete Book of Essential Oils & Aromatherapy*. Novato, Calif.: New World Library, 1991.

————. *Scents & Scentuality*. Novato, Calif.: New World Library, 1998.

Wright, Ruth V., and Robert L. Chadbourne. *Crystals, Gems and Minerals of the Bible*. New Canaan, Conn.: Keats Publishing, 1988.

Yang-Chang, Li. *Lao-Tzu's Treatise on the Response of the Tao.* New York: HarperCollins, 1994.

Yewchnode Two Wolves, Grandmother Twylah Hurd Nitsch. *Mythological Philosophy.* N.p.: private publication, 1995.

————. *The Living Circle Teaching Manual.* N.p.: private publication, 1990.

Yuthok, Dorje Yudon. *House of the Turquoise Roof.* Ithaca, N.Y.: Snow Lion, 1990.

Ziegler, John J. *Let Them Anoint the Sick.* Collegeville, Minn.: The Liturgical Press, 1987.

Acknowledgments

A book of this nature involves a great deal of research in many areas of spiritual experience. In particular I would like to thank Sheila Beber, Lita de Alberdi, Khadija, Zaneta B. Matkowska, Lily Cornford, and Maria Phylactou.

Many people within the religious community have been extremely helpful in providing me with information. I am particularly grateful to Gregorios, Archbishop of Thyateira and Great Britain, Rev. Allen Morris, Dr. Richard Mortimer, Rabbi Jonathan Magonet, Malcolm Thomas, Rev. Brian Woodock, W. Tomlinson, Richard J B Willis, Rev. Geoffrey H. Roper, Rev. David M. Chapman, Rev. A. Ward Jones, Rev. Angela Robinson, Rev. T. R. Barker, Rev. M. H. Burden, Gillian Crow, Sarah Cohen, Ani Lhamo, Andrew Fergusson, David Coffey, and Jane Clements.

Three special people were involved on this journey, and to them I am most thankful. In my search for the truth I was assisted by Julia Stonehouse, who helped me wade through the literature, and with the research into the energy of essential oils. As the fragrant threads and aromatic clues came together, we both felt the impact of inquiring into the spiritual and vibrational realms of fragrance. Lily, Julia's daughter, helped by always having the smile of innocence. And I'm grateful to my daughter, Emma, for offering her unique perspective when we experienced sweat lodges and sacred plant journeys together, and for her patience and love.

Index

𝒟

ℰ

About the Author

VALERIE ANN WORWOOD has practiced cutting-edge aromatherapy for twenty years. An aromatherapist to royalty and heads of state, she is internationally acknowledged as one of the world's leading experts in the field. Valerie lectures and conducts workshops around the world and has initiated research projects into the clinical use of essential oils. Awarded a doctorate in 1990, she has served on the executive councils of the International Federation of Aromatherapists and the Aromatherapy Organizations Council.